HEART HEALTHY
COOKBOOK FOR
BEGINNERS

600 Days of Easy and Low-Fat Time-Saving Recipes for Heart Health.
Effortlessly Achieve Lower Blood Pressure and Low Cholesterol.

By

Albert Dennison

Table of Contents

Introduction 8

What is a Heart Disease? 8

Causes and Symptoms of Heart Diseases 9

How Is Heart Disease Treated? 10

Foods To Eat 10

Food To Avoid 12

Breakfast Recipes 14

Oatmeal with Berries and Almonds 14

Avocado Toast with Whole Grain Bread 15

Greek Yogurt Parfait with Honey and Walnuts 16

Spinach and Feta Omelette 17

Chia Seed Pudding with Fresh Fruit 18

Whole Grain Pancakes with Blueberry Compote 19

Quinoa Breakfast Bowl with Mixed Nuts and Dried Fruit 21

Veggie Egg White Scramble 22

Whole Wheat Banana Nut Muffins 23

Smoked Salmon and Cream Cheese Bagel 24

Tofu Scramble with Spinach and Mushrooms 25

Cottage Cheese and Pineapple Bowl 26

Launch Recipes 28

Avocado & Black Bean Salad with Citrus Vinaigrette 28

Grilled Salmon with Lemon-Dill Sauce 29

Quinoa-Stuffed Bell Peppers 30

Mediterranean Chickpea Salad 31

Baked Chicken with Herbed Yogurt Crust 33

Spinach and Feta Stuffed Chicken Breast 34

Roasted Vegetable Tacos with Cilantro-Lime Crema 35

Whole Wheat Penne with Tomato-Basil Sauce 37

Lentil Soup with Kale and Turmeric 38

Berry-Oat Breakfast Smoothie 39

Grilled Veggie Skewers with Balsamic Glaze 40

Tofu Stir-Fry with Garlic Ginger Sauce 42

Dinner Recipes 44

Grilled Salmon with Lemon-Dill Sauce 44

Quinoa-Stuffed Bell Peppers 45

Turkey and Vegetable Stir-Fry 46

Mediterranean Chickpea Salad 48

Baked Chicken with Roasted Vegetables 49

Lentil Soup with Spinach and Tomatoes 50

Whole Wheat Pasta Primavera 51

Grilled Tofu with Garlic-Ginger Glaze 53

Spinach and Mushroom Stuffed Chicken Breast 54

Roasted Vegetable Quinoa Bowl 55

Black Bean and Corn Tacos with Avocado Salsa 56

Broiled Cod with Tomato-Caper Relish 58

Side Dish Recipes 60

Quinoa and Vegetable Salad 60

Roasted Garlic Cauliflower Mash 61

Steamed Broccoli with Lemon Garlic Sauce 62

Balsamic Glazed Brussels Sprouts..63

Spinach and Strawberry Salad 64

Herb-Roasted Sweet Potatoes 65

Grilled Asparagus with Lemon Zest 66

Lemon Herb Quinoa Pilaf 67

Roasted Beet and Arugula Salad...69

Green Bean Almondine..70

Cucumber Avocado Salad..71

Vegetable and Salad..73

Lemony Kale Salad with Avocado 73

Mediterranean Quinoa Salad with Roasted Vegetables 74

Citrus Beet and Arugula Salad 75

Grilled Vegetable Platter with Balsamic Glaze 76

Spinach and Strawberry Salad with Poppyseed Dressing 77

Roasted Cauliflower and Chickpea Salad 78

Garden Fresh Tomato and Basil Salad 80

Asian-Inspired Edamame and Cabbage Slaw 81

Roasted Sweet Potato and Brussels Sprouts Salad 82

Greek Salad with Feta and Kalamata Olives 83

Summer Corn and Black Bean Salad 84

Watermelon, Feta, and Mint Salad 86

Meat Recipes 87

Grilled Salmon with Citrus Glaze 87

Herb-Crusted Turkey Breast 88

Lemon Garlic Chicken Stir-Fry 89

Balsamic Glazed Pork Tenderloin 90

Roasted Garlic and Herb Lamb Chops 92

Turkey and Vegetable Skewers with Yogurt Sauce 93

Ginger Soy Glazed Beef Stir-Fry 95

Mediterranean Style Grilled Chicken Breast 96

Herb-Marinated Grilled Steak Salad 97

Citrus Herb Shrimp Skewers 99

Teriyaki Turkey Meatballs 100

Moroccan Spiced Chicken Tagine 101

Seafood Recipes 104

Grilled Lemon Garlic Salmon 104

Baked Herb-Crusted Tilapia 105

Seared Scallops with Citrus Salsa 106

Poached Halibut with Dill Sauce 107

Cajun Shrimp and Quinoa Salad 108

Lemon Pepper Mahi Mahi 110

Teriyaki Glazed Cod 111

Mediterranean-style Grilled Swordfish 112

Coconut Curry Shrimp Soup 113

Oven-Baked Lemon Herb Cod 115

Spicy Sriracha Tuna Lettuce Wraps 116

Grilled Shrimp and Vegetable Skewers 117

Soup and Stews Recipes 119

Lentil and Vegetable Soup 119

Quinoa and Kale Stew 120

Turkey Chili with Beans 121

Butternut Squash Soup with Ginger 123

Minestrone Soup with Whole Grain Pasta 124

Spinach and White Bean Stew 126

Chicken and Vegetable Soup with Barley 127

Moroccan Chickpea Stew 129

Tomato Basil Soup with Cannellini Beans 130

Cabbage and Potato Soup 132

Black Bean and Sweet Potato Chili 133

Lemon Chicken Orzo Soup 134

Snacks 136

Avocado and Tomato Bruschetta 136

Greek Yogurt with Honey and Almonds 137

Baked Kale Chips 138

Berry and Spinach Smoothie 139

Quinoa and Black Bean Salad Cups 140

Apple Slices with Peanut Butter and Cinnamon 141

Roasted Chickpeas with Garlic and Rosemary 142

Whole Grain Crackers with Hummus and Cherry Tomatoes 143

Steamed Edamame with Sea Salt 144

Cucumber and Feta Salad Skewers 144

Chia Seed Pudding with Mixed Berries 145

Roasted Red Pepper and White Bean Dip 146

Dessert 148

Berry Bliss Parfait 148

Avocado Chocolate Mousse 149

Lemon Chia Seed Pudding 150

Banana Oatmeal Cookies 151

Dark Chocolate-Dipped Strawberries 152

Greek Yogurt Fruit Salad 153

Almond Butter Energy Bites 154

Quinoa Berry Crumble 155

Coconut Mango Sorbet 156

Baked Apples with Cinnamon 157

Pistachio Cardamom Date Balls 158

Blueberry Oat Bars 159

Conclusion 161

Introduction

With the present state of health and fitness, individuals are seeking for strategies to preserve optimal heart and body functioning. The guidelines are intended to assist individuals in transitioning to a diet rich in fruits and vegetables, as well as lean meats and whole grains, rather than refined processed foods. According to current research, there is a strong association between blood cholesterol levels and the kind of food ingested. Low-density lipoprotein-rich foods raise blood cholesterol levels. However, dieticians and physicians have had to encourage patients to ingest high-density lipoproteins, which are beneficial fats for the body. It is vital to remember that the body still need fats; thus, you must ingest the proper sort of fats that will improve the body's functioning without raising cholesterol levels.

So, what do specialists propose in terms of heart-healthy eating? To avoid cardiovascular disease, it is advised that you follow a diet rich in low-fat dairy products, whole grains, legumes, chicken, fish, and nuts. You should restrict sugar-sweetened drinks, desserts, and red meats in your healthy diet.

Limit saturated fat consumption to 5–6% of total calorie intake.

Reduce your calorie intake of trans and saturated fats.

People who are predisposed to cardiovascular disease should limit their salt intake to less than 2300 mg to 1500 mg per day.

Limit added sugars to at least 10% of total calories ingested each day. Implementing this dietary pattern is likely to minimize your risk of cardiovascular disease. It is vital to highlight that the eating patterns in this book are not fads or diets, but rather a healthy diet plan based on scientific data to reduce the risk of chronic illnesses. It is all about the interplay of various antioxidants, minerals, vitamins, and phytochemicals that are essential for improving the activity of bodily cells. This heart-friendly cookbook has a variety of easy, nutritious, and tasty dishes, ranging from healthy breakfast options to delightful sweets. The components in this recipe are basic and readily accessible at your local grocery store. The book will help you shift your everyday eating habits in favor of healthier options.

What is a Heart Disease?

Heart disease is defined as any health condition that impairs the health or function of the heart. It is also known as cardiovascular disease, a condition that affects the heart and blood arteries. Heart disease begins with the buildup of harmful fats into the inner walls of the arteries that carry blood to our hearts. Arteriosclerosis is a disorder in which the arterial walls thicken and harden, narrowing them and restricting blood flow. As a consequence, blood cannot flow freely through these arteries, increasing the likelihood of a heart attack or stroke.

The fats accumulated in the arteries take the form of cholesterol. There are two types of cholesterol: HDL and LDL cholesterol. HDL cholesterol is healthy cholesterol; it lowers blood cholesterol levels and returns it to the liver. LDL cholesterol is dangerous because it adheres to blood arteries and may occasionally obstruct blood flow.

Causes and Symptoms of Heart Diseases

There are many causes of cardiovascular disease that affect your heart health. The causes of heart disease include.

- Born with congenital heart defects.
- Coronary artery disease is also known as blood vessel disease.
- Increased blood cholesterol.
- Family history of cardiovascular disease.
- Type-II diabetes.
- High blood pressure.

Smoking, obesity, metabolic syndrome, stress, lack of exercise, etc.

Heart disease symptoms depend on your type of CVD or

heart disease. Some of them include

Heart Arrhythmias: This is a condition in which heartbeats are abnormally fast or sluggish. Abnormal heartbeats are detected; some reasons include flapping in the chest, running heartbeats, sluggish heartbeats, near fainting, discomfort, dizziness, chest pain, and so on.

Congenital heart defects: This cardiac disease is present at birth owing to the heart's complicated anatomy. Swelling around the eye, leg, and belly are some of the symptoms and indications seen in infants. Take note of any shortness of breath or other symptoms.

Heart Cardiomyopathy: This disorder is difficult to diagnose since there are no symptoms in the early stages. When the illness progresses, symptoms include irregular heartbeats, swelling in the feet and ankles, weariness, dizziness, and lightheadedness.

Endocarditis Infection: This form of infection targets the inner lining of the heart valves and chambers. Dry cough, fever, shortness of breath, skin rashes, abnormal heart rhythm, edema, and other symptoms are signs of a heart infection.

Valvular heart disease: The heart included four valves: tricuspid, mitral, aortic, and pulmonary valves. There are many reasons of damaged heart valves. Indications and symptoms of valvular heart disease include irregular heartbeats, tiredness, chest discomfort, and fainting.

How Is Heart Disease Treated?

Lifestyle adjustments are part of the therapeutic regimen for coronary artery disease. Don't smoke. Eat lots of fruits, vegetables, and fiber-rich foods. Sugary foods should be avoided. Regular exercise is vital. Maintain a healthy weight.

Medicines: Statins are used to reduce cholesterol and treat high blood pressure. Drugs Aspirin or other blood clot-prevention drugs, diabetes medications, nitrates, beta-blockers, and other medications used to treat chest pain (angina).

Surgery: Bypass surgery, stenting (also called coronary

artery bypass grafting or CABG)

Medications Calcium channel blockers and anticoagulants are used to treat arrhythmias (blood thinners).   Ablation, cardioversion, implanted devices such as implantable cardioverter defibrillators (ICDs), and pacemakers are all viable choices.

Treatment for heart valve dysfunction includes drugs such as angiotensin-converting enzyme (ACE) inhibitors, angiotensin receptor blockers (ARBs), anti-arrhythmic medicines, antibiotics, anticoagulants (blood thinners), and beta-blockers. Diuretics Vasodilators Surgery Replacement or repair of the heart valve.

Foods To Eat

Fruits & Vegetables: These are rich in important vitamins, antioxidants, and dietary fiber. Dietary fibers assist to decrease your blood pressure and cholesterol. It also enhances blood vessel function and lowers the risk of heart disease. Seasonal fruits and vegetables are fantastic choices. Fresh fruits include potassium, magnesium, beta-carotene, and fiber.

Fruits and vegetables include:

Salads include leafy greens such spinach, lettuce, collards, Swiss chard, and kale.

Cabbage, carrots, tomatoes, cauliflower, broccoli, etc.

Fresh fruits include oranges, apples, pears, bananas, cantaloupes, papayas, and peaches. You may also use frozen, tinned, or dried fruits that have no additional sugar.

Whole Grains, cereals, and bread: Whole grains include iron, magnesium, phosphorus, vitamin B, selenium, dietary fibers, and antioxidants. Dietary fibers aid to lower blood cholesterol and excessive blood pressure. Consuming 25 grams of whole grains every day reduces the risk of heart disease by 15%. Whole grains, such as oatmeal and brown rice, aid to raise HDL levels and reduce LDL levels.

Whole grains, cereals, and bread contain:

Cereals with no added sugar, such as shredded wheat and oatmeal, are excellent options for hot and cold breakfasts.

Whole grains such as oats, millet, barley, quinoa, buckwheat, bulgur, and brown or rice are beneficial to heart health.

Whole grain bread, bagel, tortilla, and English muffins.

Fat-free or low-fat dairy products: Two servings of dairy products each day may help minimize your risk of heart disease. A fat-free dairy diet is one of the healthiest alternatives. Hemp milk contains 0mega-3 fatty acids and alpha-linolenic acid. It also includes potassium, vitamin A, vitamin D, and calcium. Dairy products contain:

- Low-fat or fat-free milk
- Soymilk, low-fat yogurt, low-fat cheese, low-fat cottage cheese, etc.

Nuts and seeds: Nuts and seeds are high in heart-healthy omega-3 fatty acids, as well as protein, fiber, vitamins, and minerals. Nuts and seeds include unsaturated fats, which assist to lower the risk of heart disease.

Nuts and seeds include:

Walnuts, peanuts, pistachios, almonds, and pecans are the finest nuts to eat for heart health.

Lean Protein: Numerous studies have shown that substituting high-fat meat with lean protein lowers blood pressure and increases good cholesterol in the body. Lean protein provides a variety of advantages, including muscle building and weight loss. Including some lean protein in your daily diet can help you stay healthy and lower your risk of heart disease.

Lean Protein includes:

- In seafood fish and shellfish,
- Poultry, turkey breast, skinless chicken, ground chicken, or turkey.
- In pork leg, tenderloin, or shoulder.
- Black beans, kidney beans, lima beans, pinto beans, chickpeas, black-eyed peas, lentils, and split peas in Beans and peas.
- Nuts, seeds, egg white, peanut butter, almond, and tofu.

Healthy oil and fats: These oils and fats are liquid at room temperature and hence better for heart health than solids. Most studies and research indicate that olive oil is one of the heart-healthy fats. It contains monounsaturated and polyunsaturated fats, as well as omega-3 fatty acids, which may help protect against heart disease. It also helps to raise the good cholesterol HDL and lower the bad cholesterol LDL levels. Trans and saturated fats are harmful fats that raise the risk of heart disease. These fats remain solid at normal temperature. Use oils in moderation.

Healthy oil and fats include:

- Vegetable oils like sunflower oil, peanut oil, safflower oil, canola oil, soybean oil, olive oil, corn oil, etc.

Food To Avoid

Excessive salt and saturated fat consumption raises blood pressure and cholesterol levels. As a result, avoid meals heavy in salt and saturated fat.

- Excess sugar in foods and drinks may elevate blood pressure and cause chronic inflammation. Excess sugar raises blood sugar levels, causes weight gain, and increases the risk of heart disease. To maintain a healthy body weight and lower your risk of heart disease, avoid eating too much sugar. Instead, add dried fruits to sweeten your meal. The American dietary standards recommend less than 10% added sugar in the daily diet.
- Avoid red and processed meats. A high diet of red meat increases your chance of developing heart disease. Eating 100g of red meat each day raises the risk of stroke and heart disease by 10-20%. Processed meat includes a lot of salt and preservatives.
- High-cholesterol foods include high-fat meats. Long-term consumption of high-cholesterol foods raises blood cholesterol and triglyceride levels. The majority of extra cholesterol accumulates within the blood vessels and arteries, reducing blood flow and increasing the risk of a heart attack or stroke. Avoid red meat (pork, steak, ribs, and beef) and processed meat (bacon, sausage, and hot dogs). Also, avoid fried foods, eggs, and seafood, which contain dangerous saturated fats.
- Processed Foods: A highly processed meal includes harmful ingredients including salt, sugar, and fat. All of these ingredients improve food flavor while increasing the risk of health problems such as obesity, high blood pressure, blood sugar levels, and heart disease. Deep-fried food, candies, sugary cereals, sweetened juices, soft drinks, margarine, cookies, and pastries are all examples of processed foods.
- Refined carbohydrates: Refined carbohydrates: are simple or bad? Carbs are rich in sugar and contribute to increased blood sugar levels. They are lacking in fiber, vitamins, and minerals, therefore refined carbohydrates are empty calories. These carbohydrates are easily digestible and have a high glycemic index. As a consequence, refined

carbohydrates cause a quick jump in blood sugar and blood insulin levels after a meal. Avoid refined carbohydrate foods including white bread, pastries, biscuits, rice cake, spaghetti, white flour, pizza dough, and morning cereals.

- Sodium (Salt): Excess salt in the diet raises blood pressure and increases the risk of cardiovascular disease. According to the American Heart Association, reducing your daily salt consumption to 1000 mg can help decrease your blood pressure. Also, always read the labels when selecting food components, and pick full, nutrient-dense foods wherever feasible.
- Excess alcohol consumption raises blood pressure and, in certain situations, causes heart failure or a stroke. Too much alcohol intake may result in abnormal heartbeats, often known as arrhythmia. Those that take alcohol do it in moderation. Females can consume one drink each day, while men can drink two.

Breakfast Recipes

Oatmeal with Berries and Almonds

Prep Time: 5 minutes
Cook Time: 10 minutes
Servings: 2

Ingredients:

- 1 cup rolled oats

- 2 cups water or milk of your choice (such as almond milk)

- 1/2 cup mixed berries (strawberries, blueberries, raspberries)

- 1/4 cup sliced almonds

- 1 tbsp. honey or maple syrup (optional)

- Pinch of cinnamon (optional)

Directions:

1. In a saucepan, heat the water or milk until it boils.

2. Stir in the oats, then decrease the heat to medium-low. Cook for 5–7 minutes, stirring periodically, until the oats are soft and creamy.

3. Remove from the heat and add the berries, almonds, and honey or maple syrup, if using.

4. Sprinkle with cinnamon if desired.

5. Divide into dishes and serve hot.

Nutrition Information (per serving):

- Calories: 250

- Total Fat: 8g

- Saturated Fat: 1g

- Cholesterol: 0mg

- Sodium: 10mg

- Total Carbohydrates: 38g

- Dietary Fiber: 7g

- Sugars: 7g

- Protein: 9g

Avocado Toast with Whole Grain Bread

Prep Time: 10 minutes
Cook Time: 5 minutes
Servings: 2

Ingredients:

- 2 slices whole grain bread

- 1 ripe avocado

- 1 tbsp. lemon juice

- Salt and pepper to taste

- Optional toppings: cherry tomatoes, red pepper flakes, sliced radishes

Directions:

1. Toast the whole-grain bread till golden brown.

2. While the bread is toasting, place the avocado flesh in a basin and mash with a fork.

3. Mix in the lemon juice, salt, and pepper.

4. Spread the mashed avocado equally over the toasted bread pieces.

5. Add extra toppings like cherry tomatoes, red pepper flakes, or sliced radishes.

6. Serve immediately.

Nutrition Information (per serving):

- Calories: 200

- Total Fat: 10g

- Saturated Fat: 1.5g

- Cholesterol: 0mg

- Sodium: 200mg

- Total Carbohydrates: 24g

- Dietary Fiber: 7g

- Sugars: 2g

- Protein: 5g

Greek Yogurt Parfait with Honey and Walnuts

Prep Time: 5 minutes
Servings: 2

Ingredients:

- 1 cup Greek yogurt

- 2 tbsp. honey

- 1/4 cup chopped walnuts

- 1/2 cup mixed berries (strawberries, blueberries, raspberries)

- 1/4 cup granola (optional)

Directions:

1. In two serving glasses or bowls, arrange Greek yogurt, mixed berries, and chopped walnuts.

2. Drizzle each layer with honey.

3. Repeat the layers until the glasses are full.

4. Top with granola for extra crunch.

5. Serve immediately for a tasty and healthful breakfast or snack.

Nutrition Information (per serving):

- Calories: 250

- Total Fat: 12g

- Saturated Fat: 1.5g

- Cholesterol: 10mg

- Sodium: 40mg

- Total Carbohydrates: 25g

- Dietary Fiber: 3g

- Sugars: 18g

- Protein: 15g

Spinach and Feta Omelette

Prep Time: 5 minutes
Cook Time: 5 minutes
Servings: 2

Ingredients:

- 4 large eggs

- 2 cups fresh spinach leaves

- 1/4 cup crumbled feta cheese

- Salt and pepper to taste

- 1 tbsp. olive oil

Directions:

1. In a mixing basin, whisk together the eggs until thoroughly combined. Season with salt and pepper.

2. In a nonstick skillet, heat olive oil over medium heat.

3. Cook the spinach leaves in the pan for 1-2 minutes, or until wilted.

4. Pour the beaten eggs over the spinach and swirl the pan to distribute them evenly.

5. Cook for 2-3 minutes, until the edges are set.

6. Sprinkle the crumbled feta cheese on one side of the omelette.

7. Using a spatula, fold the remaining half of the omelette over the cheese.

8. Cook for a further 1-2 minutes, or until the cheese has melted and the omelette is fully cooked.

9. Transfer the omelette to a platter and serve hot.

Nutrition Information (per serving):

- Calories: 220

- Total Fat: 17g

- Saturated Fat: 5g

- Cholesterol: 380mg

- Sodium: 380mg

- Total Carbohydrates: 3g

- Dietary Fiber: 1g

- Sugars: 1g

- Protein: 14g

Chia Seed Pudding with Fresh Fruit

Prep Time: 5 minutes (plus chilling time)
Servings: 2

Ingredients:

- 1/4 cup chia seeds

- 1 cup unsweetened almond milk (or any milk of your choice)

- 1 tbsp. honey or maple syrup (optional)

- 1/2 tsp. vanilla extract

- Fresh fruit of your choice for topping (e.g., strawberries, blueberries, raspberries)

Directions:

1. In a bowl, combine the chia seeds, almond milk, honey or maple syrup (if using), and vanilla essence.

2. Stir until thoroughly combined and free of clumps.

3. Cover and refrigerate for at least 2 hours, or overnight, until the liquid thickens to a pudding consistency.

4. Serve topped with fresh fruit.

Nutrition Information (per serving):

- Calories: 150

- Total Fat: 8g

- Saturated Fat: 1g

- Cholesterol: 0mg

- Sodium: 80mg

- Total Carbohydrates: 15g

- Dietary Fiber: 8g

- Sugars: 5g

- Protein: 5g

Whole Grain Pancakes with Blueberry Compote

Prep Time: 10 minutes
Cook Time: 15 minutes
Servings: 4

Ingredients:

For Pancakes:

- 1 cup whole wheat flour

- 1 tbsp. baking powder

- 1 tbsp. honey or maple syrup

- 1 cup milk (dairy or plant-based)

- 1 egg

- 1 tbsp. melted butter or oil

- Pinch of salt

For Blueberry Compote:

- 1 cup fresh or frozen blueberries

- 2 tbsp. water

- 1 tbsp. honey or maple syrup

Directions:

For Pancakes:

1. In a large bowl, combine the flour, baking powder, and salt.

2. In a separate dish, mix together the honey or maple syrup, milk, egg, and melted butter or oil.

3. Pour the wet ingredients into the dry ingredients and mix just until mixed.

4. Cook on a lightly greased pan or griddle over medium-high heat.

5. Pour about 1/4 cup batter onto the skillet for each pancake.

6. Cook until bubbles appear on the top, then turn and cook until golden brown on the other side.

7. Repeat with the remaining batter.

For Blueberry Compote:

1. In a small saucepan, mix the blueberries, water, and honey/maple syrup.

2. Bring to a simmer over medium heat, stirring regularly, for approximately 5 minutes, or until the blueberries have broken down and the sauce thickens somewhat.

3. Remove from heat and let it cool slightly before serving with pancakes.

Nutrition Information (per serving, including compote):

- Calories: 280
- Total Fat: 6g
- Saturated Fat: 2g
- Cholesterol: 45mg
- Sodium: 320mg
- Total Carbohydrates: 50g
- Dietary Fiber: 6g
- Sugars: 15g
- Protein: 9g

Quinoa Breakfast Bowl with Mixed Nuts and Dried Fruit

Prep Time: 5 minutes
Cook Time: 15 minutes
Servings: 2

Ingredients:

- 1/2 cup quinoa, rinsed
- 1 cup water or milk (dairy or plant-based)
- 1/4 cup mixed nuts (such as almonds, walnuts, pistachios)
- 1/4 cup dried fruit (such as raisins, cranberries, apricots)
- 1 tbsp. honey or maple syrup (optional)
- Pinch of cinnamon (optional)

Directions:

1. In a saucepan, mix the quinoa and water or milk.
2. Bring to a boil, then lower to a low heat, cover, and simmer for 15 minutes, or until the quinoa is cooked and the liquid has been absorbed.
3. Fluff the quinoa with a fork and divide it into bowls.
4. Top with a mixture of nuts and dried fruit, then drizzle with honey or maple syrup as preferred.
5. If using, sprinkle with cinnamon.
6. Serve warm.

Nutrition Information (per serving):

- Calories: 300
- Total Fat: 10g
- Saturated Fat: 1g
- Cholesterol: 0mg
- Sodium: 10mg
- Total Carbohydrates: 45g
- Dietary Fiber: 6g

- Sugars: 15g

- Protein: 9g

Veggie Egg White Scramble

Prep Time: 5 minutes
Cook Time: 5 minutes
Servings: 2

Ingredients:

- 4 large egg whites

- 1/2 cup diced mixed vegetables (such as bell peppers, onions, spinach)

- 1 tbsp. olive oil

- Salt and pepper to taste

- Optional: chopped fresh herbs (such as parsley or chives)

Directions:

1. In a nonstick skillet, heat olive oil over medium heat.

2. Sauté the diced veggies for 2-3 minutes, until softened.

3. Add the egg whites and season with salt and pepper.

4. Cook, stirring periodically, until the egg whites have set and scrambled.

5. Sprinkle with chopped fresh herbs, if desired.

6. Serve hot.

Nutrition Information (per serving):

- Calories: 70

- Total Fat: 4g

- Saturated Fat: 0.5g

- Cholesterol: 0mg

- Sodium: 150mg

- Total Carbohydrates: 4g

- Dietary Fiber: 1g

- Sugars: 2g

- Protein: 5g

Whole Wheat Banana Nut Muffins

Prep Time: 15 minutes
Cook Time: 20 minutes
Servings: 12

Ingredients:

- 1 1/2 cups whole wheat flour

- 1 tsp. baking powder

- 1/2 tsp. baking soda

- 1/4 tsp. salt

- 3 ripe bananas, mashed

- 1/4 cup honey or maple syrup

- 1/4 cup plain Greek yogurt

- 1/4 cup unsweetened applesauce

- 1 egg

- 1 tsp. vanilla extract

- 1/2 cup chopped walnuts or pecans (optional)

Directions:

1. Preheat the oven to 350° Fahrenheit (175° Celsius). Line a muffin tray with paper liners or spray with cooking spray.

2. In a large basin, combine the flour, baking powder, baking soda, and salt.

3. In another dish, add the mashed bananas, honey or maple syrup, Greek yogurt, applesauce, egg, and vanilla extract.

4. Pour the wet ingredients into the dry ingredients and mix just until mixed. Fold in the chopped nuts, if using.

5. Divide the batter equally into the muffin cups.

6. Bake for 18 to 20 minutes, or until a toothpick inserted in the middle comes out clean.

7. Allow muffins to cool in their tins for 5 minutes before transferring to a wire rack to finish cooling.

Nutrition Information (per muffin):

- Calories: 150
- Total Fat: 4g
- Saturated Fat: 0.5g
- Cholesterol: 15mg
- Sodium: 140mg
- Total Carbohydrates: 27g
- Dietary Fiber: 3g
- Sugars: 12g
- Protein: 4g

Smoked Salmon and Cream Cheese Bagel

Prep Time: 5 minutes
Servings: 1

Ingredients:

- 1 whole wheat bagel, sliced and toasted
- 2 tbsp. reduced-fat cream cheese
- 2 oz. smoked salmon
- Sliced cucumber, red onion, and capers for garnish (optional)
- Fresh dill or chives for garnish (optional)

Directions:

1. Spread the cream cheese equally over both half of the toasted bagel.

2. Place smoked salmon on top of the cream cheese.

3. Garnish with sliced cucumber, red onion, capers, and fresh dill or chives if preferred.

4. Serve immediately.

Nutrition Information (per serving):

- Calories: 370

- Total Fat: 11g

- Saturated Fat: 4.5g

- Cholesterol: 40mg

- Sodium: 860mg

- Total Carbohydrates: 44g

- Dietary Fiber: 6g

- Sugars: 6g

- Protein: 24g

Tofu Scramble with Spinach and Mushrooms

Prep Time: 10 minutes
Cook Time: 10 minutes
Servings: 2

Ingredients:

- 1 tbsp. olive oil

- 8 oz. firm tofu, drained and crumbled

- 1 cup sliced mushrooms

- 2 cups fresh spinach leaves

- 1/2 tsp. turmeric powder

- Salt and pepper to taste

Directions:

1. In a medium-size pan, heat the olive oil.

2. Add the crumbled tofu and sliced mushrooms to the skillet. Cook 5 minutes, stirring periodically.

3. Add the fresh spinach leaves and turmeric powder to the skillet. Cook for a further 2-3 minutes until the spinach has wilted.

4. Season with salt and pepper to taste.

5. Serve hot.

Nutrition Information (per serving):

- Calories: 180
- Total Fat: 13g
- Saturated Fat: 2g
- Cholesterol: 0mg
- Sodium: 80mg
- Total Carbohydrates: 7g
- Dietary Fiber: 3g
- Sugars: 2g
- Protein: 12g

Cottage Cheese and Pineapple Bowl

Prep Time: 5 minutes
Servings: 1

Ingredients:

- 1/2 cup low-fat cottage cheese
- 1/2 cup diced fresh pineapple
- 1 tbsp. chopped walnuts or almonds (optional)
- 1 tsp. honey (optional)

Directions:

1. In a bowl, combine cottage cheese and diced pineapple.

2. If desired, sprinkle with chopped nuts and drizzle with honey.

3. Serve chilled.

Nutrition Information (per serving):

- Calories: 180
- Total Fat: 4g
- Saturated Fat: 0.5g
- Cholesterol: 5mg
- Sodium: 400mg
- Total Carbohydrates: 21g
- Dietary Fiber: 2g
- Sugars: 16g
- Protein: 16g

Launch Recipes

Avocado & Black Bean Salad with Citrus Vinaigrette

Prep Time: 15 minutes
Servings: 4

Ingredients:

- 2 ripe avocados, diced
- 1 can (15 oz) black beans, rinsed and drained
- 1 cup cherry tomatoes, halved
- 1/4 cup red onion, finely chopped
- 1/4 cup cilantro, chopped
- Juice of 1 lime
- 2 tbsp. orange juice
- 1 tbsp. olive oil
- Salt and pepper to taste

Directions:

1. In a large mixing dish, add chopped avocado, black beans, cherry tomatoes, red onion, and cilantro.
2. In a small mixing bowl, combine the lime juice, orange juice, olive oil, salt, and pepper to create the vinaigrette.
3. Pour the vinaigrette over the salad and toss to coat.
4. Serve cold.

Nutrition Information (per serving):

- Calories: 250
- Total Fat: 12g
- Saturated Fat: 1.5g
- Cholesterol: 0mg

- Sodium: 250mg

- Total Carbohydrates: 32g

- Dietary Fiber: 12g

- Sugars: 3g

- Protein: 9g

Grilled Salmon with Lemon-Dill Sauce

Prep Time: 10 minutes
Cook Time: 10 minutes
Servings: 4

Ingredients:

- 4 salmon fillets

- 2 tbsp. olive oil

- Salt and pepper to taste

- Lemon wedges for serving

For Lemon-Dill Sauce:

- 1/4 cup plain Greek yogurt

- 1 tbsp. chopped fresh dill

- 1 tbsp. lemon juice

- Salt and pepper to taste

Directions:

1. Preheat the grill for medium-high heat.

2. Brush olive oil over salmon fillets and season with salt and pepper.

3. Grill salmon for 4-5 minutes each side, or until cooked through.

4. Meanwhile, in a separate bowl, combine the Greek yogurt, chopped dill, lemon juice, salt, and pepper to prepare the sauce.

5. Serve grilled salmon with lemon wedges and a lemon-dill sauce.

Nutrition Information (per serving):

- Calories: 300

- Total Fat: 18g

- Saturated Fat: 3.5g

- Cholesterol: 80mg

- Sodium: 70mg

- Total Carbohydrates: 2g

- Dietary Fiber: 0g

- Sugars: 1g

- Protein: 32g

Quinoa-Stuffed Bell Peppers

Prep Time: 15 minutes
Cook Time: 30 minutes
Servings: 4

Ingredients:

- 4 bell peppers, halved and seeds removed

- 1 cup cooked quinoa

- 1 can (15 oz) black beans, rinsed and drained

- 1 cup corn kernels

- 1 cup diced tomatoes

- 1/2 cup diced red onion

- 1/4 cup chopped cilantro

- 1 tsp. ground cumin

- 1/2 tsp. chili powder

- Salt and pepper to taste

- 1/2 cup shredded cheddar cheese (optional)

Directions:

1. Preheat the oven to 375° Fahrenheit (190° Celsius). Arrange the bell pepper halves in a baking dish.

2. In a large mixing bowl, add the cooked quinoa, black beans, corn kernels, diced tomatoes, red onion, cilantro, cumin, chili powder, salt, and pepper.

3. Spoon the quinoa mixture into each bell pepper half until completely filled.

4. Cover the baking dish with foil and bake for 25-30 minutes, until the peppers are cooked.

5. If preferred, top the filled peppers with shredded cheddar cheese during the final 5 minutes of baking.

6. Serve hot.

Nutrition Information (per serving):

- Calories: 250
- Total Fat: 3.5g
- Saturated Fat: 1g
- Cholesterol: 5mg
- Sodium: 260mg
- Total Carbohydrates: 45g
- Dietary Fiber: 11g
- Sugars: 7g
- Protein: 12g

Mediterranean Chickpea Salad

Prep Time: 10 minutes
Servings: 4

Ingredients:

- 1 can (15 oz) chickpeas, rinsed and drained
- 1 cup diced cucumber
- 1 cup cherry tomatoes, halved

- 1/2 cup diced red onion

- 1/4 cup chopped fresh parsley

- 1/4 cup crumbled feta cheese

- 2 tbsp. extra virgin olive oil

- 1 tbsp. lemon juice

- 1 tsp. dried oregano

- Salt and pepper to taste

Directions:

1. In a large mixing basin, add chickpeas, cucumber, cherry tomatoes, red onion, parsley, and feta cheese.

2. Make the dressing by whisking together olive oil, lemon juice, dried oregano, salt, and pepper in a small bowl.

3. Pour the dressing over the salad and toss to coat evenly.

4. Serve cold.

Nutrition Information (per serving):

- Calories: 220

- Total Fat: 11g

- Saturated Fat: 2.5g

- Cholesterol: 10mg

- Sodium: 250mg

- Total Carbohydrates: 25g

- Dietary Fiber: 6g

- Sugars: 5g

- Protein: 8g

Baked Chicken with Herbed Yogurt Crust

Prep Time: 10 minutes
Cook Time: 25 minutes
Servings: 4

Ingredients:

- 4 boneless, skinless chicken breasts
- 1 cup plain Greek yogurt
- 2 cloves garlic, minced
- 2 tbsp. chopped fresh herbs (such as parsley, thyme, rosemary)
- 1 tbsp. lemon juice
- Salt and pepper to taste

Directions:

1. Preheat the oven to 400 °F (200 °C). Lightly oil a baking dish.
2. In a bowl, combine Greek yogurt, minced garlic, chopped fresh herbs, lemon juice, salt, and pepper.
3. Place the chicken breasts in the prepared baking dish.
4. Spread the herbed yogurt mixture equally on top of each chicken breast.
5. Bake for 20-25 minutes, or until the chicken is well cooked and the crust is golden brown.
6. Serve hot.

Nutrition Information (per serving):

- Calories: 200
- Total Fat: 4g
- Saturated Fat: 1g
- Cholesterol: 85mg
- Sodium: 120mg
- Total Carbohydrates: 2g
- Dietary Fiber: 0g

- Sugars: 1g

- Protein: 38g

Spinach and Feta Stuffed Chicken Breast

Prep Time: 15 minutes
Cook Time: 25 minutes
Servings: 4

Ingredients:

- 4 boneless, skinless chicken breasts

- 2 cups fresh spinach leaves

- 1/2 cup crumbled feta cheese

- 2 cloves garlic, minced

- 1 tbsp. olive oil

- Salt and pepper to taste

Directions:

1. Preheat the oven to 375° Fahrenheit (190° Celsius). Lightly oil a baking dish.

2. In a pan, heat the olive oil over medium heat. Cook for approximately 1 minute, or until the garlic is aromatic.

3. Cook the fresh spinach leaves in the pan until wilted, approximately 2-3 minutes. Remove from heat and let it cool slightly.

4. Create a pocket in each chicken breast, taking care not to cut all the way through.

5. Fill each chicken breast with wilted spinach and crumbled feta.

6. Season the filled chicken breasts with salt and pepper.

7. Place the filled chicken breasts in the prepared baking dish.

8. Bake for 20-25 minutes, or until the chicken is cooked through.

9. Serve hot.

Nutrition Information (per serving):

- Calories: 250

- Total Fat: 9g

- Saturated Fat: 3g

- Cholesterol: 100mg

- Sodium: 300mg

- Total Carbohydrates: 2g

- Dietary Fiber: 1g

- Sugars: 0g

- Protein: 38g

Roasted Vegetable Tacos with Cilantro-Lime Crema

Prep Time: 15 minutes
Cook Time: 25 minutes
Servings: 4

Ingredients:

For Roasted Vegetables:

- 2 bell peppers, sliced

- 1 red onion, sliced

- 1 zucchini, sliced

- 1 tbsp. olive oil

- 1 tsp. ground cumin

- 1 tsp. chili powder

- Salt and pepper to taste

For Cilantro-Lime Crema:

- 1/2 cup plain Greek yogurt

- 2 tbsp. chopped fresh cilantro

- 1 tbsp. lime juice

- Salt to taste

For Tacos:

- 8 small whole wheat tortillas
- Additional toppings such as avocado slices, shredded lettuce, diced tomatoes

Directions:

For Roasted Vegetables:

1. Preheat the oven to 400 °F (200 °C). Line a baking sheet with parchment paper.
2. In a large mixing bowl, combine sliced bell peppers, red onion, zucchini, olive oil, ground cumin, chili powder, salt, and pepper.
3. Place the seasoned veggies in a single layer on the prepared baking sheet.
4. Roast in a preheated oven for 20-25 minutes, or until the veggies are soft and faintly caramelized.

For Cilantro-Lime Crema:

1. In a small bowl, combine the Greek yogurt, chopped cilantro, lime juice, and salt to taste. Adjust the seasoning as needed.

Assembling Tacos:

1. Warm the whole wheat tortillas according to the package directions.
2. Fill each tortilla with roasted veggies, then top with cilantro-lime crema.
3. If preferred, add avocado slices, shredded lettuce, or sliced tomatoes.
4. Serve immediately.

Nutrition Information (per serving, including 2 tacos):

- Calories: 300
- Total Fat: 9g
- Saturated Fat: 1.5g
- Cholesterol: 5mg
- Sodium: 350mg
- Total Carbohydrates: 45g
- Dietary Fiber: 9g
- Sugars: 5g

- Protein: 12g

Whole Wheat Penne with Tomato-Basil Sauce

Prep Time: 10 minutes
Cook Time: 20 minutes
Servings: 4

Ingredients:

- 8 oz whole wheat penne pasta
- 2 tbsp. olive oil
- 2 cloves garlic, minced
- 1 can (14.5 oz) diced tomatoes
- 1/4 cup tomato paste
- 1 tsp. dried oregano
- 1 tsp. dried basil
- Salt and pepper to taste
- Fresh basil leaves for garnish
- Grated Parmesan cheese for serving (optional)

Directions:

1. Cook the whole wheat penne pasta according to the package directions until al dente. Drain and put aside.

2. In a large skillet, heat the olive oil over medium heat. Sauté minced garlic until fragrant, approximately 1 minute.

3. Add diced tomatoes (with juices), tomato paste, dry oregano, and dried basil to the skillet. Season with salt and pepper to taste.

4. Simmer the sauce for 10-15 minutes, stirring regularly, until it has thickened somewhat.

5. Toss the cooked penne pasta in the pan with the tomato-basil sauce until evenly coated.

6. Garnish with fresh basil leaves.

7. If preferred, serve hot with grated Parmesan cheese.

Nutrition Information (per serving):

- Calories: 300
- Total Fat: 7g
- Saturated Fat: 1g
- Cholesterol: 0mg
- Sodium: 200mg
- Total Carbohydrates: 52g
- Dietary Fiber: 8g
- Sugars: 6g
- Protein: 10g

Lentil Soup with Kale and Turmeric

Prep Time: 10 minutes
Cook Time: 30 minutes
Servings: 6

Ingredients:

- 1 tbsp. olive oil
- 1 onion, diced
- 2 carrots, diced
- 2 celery stalks, diced
- 2 cloves garlic, minced
- 1 cup dried green lentils, rinsed
- 6 cups vegetable broth
- 2 cups chopped kale leaves
- 1 tsp. ground turmeric
- Salt and pepper to taste
- Fresh lemon wedges for serving

Directions:

1. In a large saucepan, heat the olive oil over medium heat. Add the diced onions, carrots, and celery. Sauté the veggies for approximately 5 minutes, or until tender.

2. Add the minced garlic and cook for another minute, or until fragrant.

3. Add the dry green lentils and vegetable broth to the saucepan. Bring to a boil, then lower to a low heat and cook for 20-25 minutes, until lentils are cooked.

4. Stir in the chopped kale leaves and ground turmeric. Cook for a further 5 minutes, until the kale has wilted.

5. Season with salt and pepper to taste.

6. Serve hot, with fresh lemon wedges to squeeze over the soup.

Nutrition Information (per serving):

- Calories: 200
- Total Fat: 3g
- Saturated Fat: 0g
- Cholesterol: 0mg
- Sodium: 600mg
- Total Carbohydrates: 32g
- Dietary Fiber: 12g
- Sugars: 5g
- Protein: 11g

Berry-Oat Breakfast Smoothie

Prep Time: 5 minutes
Servings: 2

Ingredients:

- 1 cup mixed berries (such as strawberries, blueberries, raspberries)
- 1 ripe banana
- 1/2 cup rolled oats

- 1 cup unsweetened almond milk (or any milk of your choice)

- 1 tbsp. honey or maple syrup (optional)

- Ice cubes (optional)

Directions:

1. In a blender, combine mixed berries, ripe banana, rolled oats, almond milk, and honey or maple syrup (if desired).

2. Blend until smooth and creamy.

3. If required, add more ice cubes and mix until smooth.

4. Pour into glasses and serve immediately.

Nutrition Information (per serving):

- Calories: 200

- Total Fat: 3g

- Saturated Fat: 0g

- Cholesterol: 0mg

- Sodium: 100mg

- Total Carbohydrates: 42g

- Dietary Fiber: 7g

- Sugars: 18g

- Protein: 5g

Grilled Veggie Skewers with Balsamic Glaze

Prep Time: 15 minutes
Cook Time: 10 minutes
Servings: 4

Ingredients:

- 2 bell peppers, cut into chunks

- 1 zucchini, sliced

- 1 yellow squash, sliced

- 1 red onion, cut into chunks
- 8 cherry tomatoes
- 8 cremini mushrooms
- 2 tbsp. olive oil
- Salt and pepper to taste
- Balsamic glaze for drizzling
- Fresh parsley for garnish (optional)

Directions:

1. Preheat the grill for medium-high heat.
2. Thread skewers with bell pepper, zucchini, yellow squash, red onion, cherry tomatoes, and cremini mushrooms.
3. Brush the skewered veggies with olive oil and season with salt and pepper.
4. Grill the vegetable skewers for 8-10 minutes, rotating periodically, until soft and gently browned.
5. Transfer the grilled vegetable skewers to a serving plate.
6. Drizzle with balsamic glaze and serve with fresh parsley, if preferred.
7. Serve hot.

Nutrition Information (per serving):

- Calories: 120
- Total Fat: 7g
- Saturated Fat: 1g
- Cholesterol: 0mg
- Sodium: 20mg
- Total Carbohydrates: 14g
- Dietary Fiber: 4g
- Sugars: 8g
- Protein: 3g

Tofu Stir-Fry with Garlic Ginger Sauce

Prep Time: 15 minutes
Cook Time: 15 minutes
Servings: 4

Ingredients:

- 14 oz firm tofu, pressed and cubed
- 2 tbsp. soy sauce
- 1 tbsp. rice vinegar
- 1 tbsp. honey or maple syrup
- 2 cloves garlic, minced
- 1 tsp. grated ginger
- 1 tbsp. cornstarch
- 2 tbsp. water
- 2 tbsp. sesame oil
- 1 bell pepper, sliced
- 1 cup broccoli florets
- 1 carrot, sliced
- Cooked brown rice for serving

Directions:

1. In a mixing bowl, combine soy sauce, rice vinegar, honey or maple syrup, chopped garlic, and grated ginger to create the sauce.

2. In another small bowl, combine cornstarch and water to produce a slurry.

3. Heat the sesame oil in a large pan or wok over medium-high heat.

4. Cook cubed tofu in the skillet until golden brown on both sides, approximately 5-7 minutes. Remove the tofu from the skillet and put aside.

5. In the same pan, combine sliced bell pepper, broccoli florets, and sliced carrot. Stir-fry for 3-4 minutes, until the veggies are crisp-tender.

6. Return the tofu to the skillet. Pour the sauce over the tofu and veggies.

7. Add the cornstarch slurry and boil for another 2-3 minutes, or until the sauce thickens.

8. Serve the tofu stir-fry over cooked brown rice.

Nutrition Information (per serving, tofu stir-fry only, without rice):

- Calories: 180
- Total Fat: 12g
- Saturated Fat: 2g
- Cholesterol: 0mg
- Sodium: 450mg
- Total Carbohydrates: 11g
- Dietary Fiber: 3g
- Sugars: 5g
- Protein: 10g

Grilled Salmon with Lemon-Dill Sauce

Prep Time: 10 minutes
Cook Time: 10 minutes
Servings: 4

Ingredients:

- 4 salmon fillets
- 2 tbsp. olive oil
- Salt and pepper to taste
- Lemon wedges for serving

For Lemon-Dill Sauce:

- 1/4 cup plain Greek yogurt
- 1 tbsp. chopped fresh dill
- 1 tbsp. lemon juice
- Salt and pepper to taste

Directions:

1. Preheat the grill for medium-high heat.
2. Brush olive oil over salmon fillets and season with salt and pepper.
3. Grill salmon for 4-5 minutes each side, or until cooked through.
4. Meanwhile, in a separate bowl, combine the Greek yogurt, chopped dill, lemon juice, salt, and pepper to prepare the sauce.
5. Serve grilled salmon with lemon wedges and a lemon-dill sauce.

Nutrition Information (per serving):

- Calories: 250
- Total Fat: 15g
- Saturated Fat: 2.5g

- Cholesterol: 70mg

- Sodium: 100mg

- Total Carbohydrates: 1g

- Dietary Fiber: 0g

- Sugars: 0g

- Protein: 25g

Quinoa-Stuffed Bell Peppers

Prep Time: 15 minutes
Cook Time: 30 minutes
Servings: 4

Ingredients:

- 4 bell peppers, halved and seeds removed

- 1 cup cooked quinoa

- 1 can (15 oz) black beans, rinsed and drained

- 1 cup corn kernels

- 1 cup diced tomatoes

- 1/2 cup diced red onion

- 1/4 cup chopped cilantro

- 1 tsp. ground cumin

- 1/2 tsp. chili powder

- Salt and pepper to taste

- 1/2 cup shredded cheddar cheese (optional)

Directions:

1. Preheat the oven to 375° Fahrenheit (190° Celsius). Arrange the bell pepper halves in a baking dish.

2. In a large mixing bowl, add the cooked quinoa, black beans, corn kernels, diced tomatoes, red onion, cilantro, cumin, chili powder, salt, and pepper.

3. Spoon the quinoa mixture into each bell pepper half until completely filled.

4. Cover the baking dish with foil and bake for 25-30 minutes, until the peppers are cooked.

5. If preferred, top the filled peppers with shredded cheddar cheese during the final 5 minutes of baking.

6. Serve hot.

Nutrition Information (per serving):

- Calories: 300
- Total Fat: 3.5g
- Saturated Fat: 1g
- Cholesterol: 5mg
- Sodium: 260mg
- Total Carbohydrates: 45g
- Dietary Fiber: 11g
- Sugars: 7g
- Protein: 12g

Turkey and Vegetable Stir-Fry

Prep Time: 15 minutes
Cook Time: 15 minutes
Servings: 4

Ingredients:

- 1 lb turkey breast, sliced into thin strips
- 2 tbsp. soy sauce
- 1 tbsp. rice vinegar
- 1 tbsp. honey or maple syrup
- 1 tbsp. sesame oil
- 2 cloves garlic, minced

- 1 tbsp. grated ginger
- 1 bell pepper, sliced
- 1 cup broccoli florets
- 1 carrot, sliced
- 1 cup snap peas
- Cooked brown rice for serving

Directions:

1. In a mixing bowl, combine soy sauce, rice vinegar, honey or maple syrup, sesame oil, chopped garlic, and grated ginger to create the sauce.
2. Preheat a big pan or wok to medium-high heat. Stir-fry the turkey breast strips for 5-6 minutes, or until well done. Remove from the skillet and put aside.
3. In the same pan, combine the sliced bell pepper, broccoli florets, sliced carrot, and snap peas. Stir-fry for 4-5 minutes, until the veggies are crisp-tender.
4. Return the cooked turkey breast strips to the skillet. Pour the sauce over the turkey and veggies.
5. Stir-fry for a further 2-3 minutes, or until everything is well cooked and covered with sauce.
6. Serve the turkey and veggie stir fry over cooked brown rice.

Nutrition Information (per serving, stir-fry only, without rice):

- Calories: 200
- Total Fat: 5g
- Saturated Fat: 1g
- Cholesterol: 65mg
- Sodium: 450mg
- Total Carbohydrates: 15g
- Dietary Fiber: 3g
- Sugars: 8g
- Protein: 25g

Mediterranean Chickpea Salad

Prep Time: 10 minutes
Servings: 4

Ingredients:

- 1 can (15 oz) chickpeas, rinsed and drained
- 1 cup diced cucumber
- 1 cup cherry tomatoes, halved
- 1/2 cup diced red onion
- 1/4 cup chopped fresh parsley
- 1/4 cup crumbled feta cheese
- 2 tbsp. extra virgin olive oil
- 1 tbsp. lemon juice
- 1 tsp. dried oregano
- Salt and pepper to taste

Directions:

1. In a large mixing basin, add chickpeas, cucumber, cherry tomatoes, red onion, parsley, and feta cheese.
2. Make the dressing by whisking together olive oil, lemon juice, dried oregano, salt, and pepper in a small bowl.
3. Pour the dressing over the salad and toss to coat evenly.
4. Serve cold.

Nutrition Information (per serving):

- Calories: 220
- Total Fat: 11g
- Saturated Fat: 2.5g
- Cholesterol: 10mg
- Sodium: 250mg

- Total Carbohydrates: 25g

- Dietary Fiber: 6g

- Sugars: 5g

- Protein: 8g

Baked Chicken with Roasted Vegetables

Prep Time: 15 minutes
Cook Time: 30 minutes
Servings: 4

Ingredients:

- 4 boneless, skinless chicken breasts

- 2 tbsp. olive oil

- 1 tsp. dried thyme

- 1 tsp. dried rosemary

- Salt and pepper to taste

- 2 cups mixed vegetables (such as carrots, bell peppers, zucchini, cherry tomatoes)

- 1 tbsp. balsamic vinegar

Directions:

1. Preheat the oven to 400 °F (200 °C). Lightly oil a baking dish.

2. Place the chicken breasts in the prepared baking dish. Drizzle with olive oil, then sprinkle with dried thyme, rosemary, salt, and pepper.

3. In a separate dish, combine the veggies with olive oil, salt, pepper, and balsamic vinegar.

4. Arrange the mixed veggies around the chicken breasts in the baking dish.

5. Bake for 25-30 minutes, or until the chicken is fully cooked and the veggies are soft.

6. Serve hot.

Nutrition Information (per serving):

- Calories: 250

- Total Fat: 10g

- Saturated Fat: 1.5g

- Cholesterol: 70mg

- Sodium: 120mg

- Total Carbohydrates: 8g

- Dietary Fiber: 2g

- Sugars: 4g

- Protein: 30g

Lentil Soup with Spinach and Tomatoes

Prep Time: 10 minutes
Cook Time: 30 minutes
Servings: 6

Ingredients:

- 1 tbsp. olive oil

- 1 onion, diced

- 2 carrots, diced

- 2 celery stalks, diced

- 2 cloves garlic, minced

- 1 cup dried green lentils, rinsed

- 6 cups vegetable broth

- 2 cups chopped spinach leaves

- 1 can (14.5 oz) diced tomatoes

- 1 tsp. dried thyme

- Salt and pepper to taste

Directions:

1. In a large saucepan, heat the olive oil over medium heat. Add the diced onions, carrots, and celery. Sauté the veggies for approximately 5 minutes, or until tender.

2. Add the minced garlic and cook for another minute, or until fragrant.

3. Add the dry green lentils and vegetable broth to the saucepan. Bring to a boil, then lower to a low heat and cook for 20-25 minutes, until lentils are cooked.

4. Stir in the chopped spinach leaves, diced tomatoes (with juices), and dried thyme. Simmer for a further 5 minutes.

5. Season with salt and pepper to taste.

6. Serve hot.

Nutrition Information (per serving):

- Calories: 200

- Total Fat: 3g

- Saturated Fat: 0g

- Cholesterol: 0mg

- Sodium: 600mg

- Total Carbohydrates: 32g

- Dietary Fiber: 12g

- Sugars: 5g

- Protein: 11g

Whole Wheat Pasta Primavera

Prep Time: 10 minutes
Cook Time: 15 minutes
Servings: 4

Ingredients:

- 8 oz whole wheat spaghetti

- 2 tbsp. olive oil

- 2 cloves garlic, minced

- 1 cup cherry tomatoes, halved

- 1 cup broccoli florets

- 1 cup sliced bell peppers

- 1 cup sliced zucchini

- 1/4 cup chopped fresh basil

- Salt and pepper to taste

- Grated Parmesan cheese for serving (optional)

Directions:

1. Cook whole wheat spaghetti according to the package directions until al dente. Drain and put aside.

2. In a large skillet, heat the olive oil over medium heat. Sauté minced garlic until fragrant, approximately 1 minute.

3. Add the cherry tomatoes, broccoli florets, sliced bell peppers, and sliced zucchini to the pan. Stir-fry for 4-5 minutes, until the veggies are crisp-tender.

4. Add the cooked whole wheat spaghetti to the skillet. Toss to evenly coat the veggies.

5. Stir in the chopped fresh basil. Season with salt and pepper to taste.

6. If preferred, serve hot with grated Parmesan cheese.

Nutrition Information (per serving):

- Calories: 300

- Total Fat: 9g

- Saturated Fat: 1.5g

- Cholesterol: 0mg

- Sodium: 20mg

- Total Carbohydrates: 45g

- Dietary Fiber: 9g

- Sugars: 6g

- Protein: 10g

Grilled Tofu with Garlic-Ginger Glaze

Prep Time: 15 minutes
Cook Time: 10 minutes
Servings: 4

Ingredients:

- 14 oz firm tofu, pressed and sliced into rectangles
- 2 tbsp. soy sauce
- 1 tbsp. rice vinegar
- 1 tbsp. honey or maple syrup
- 2 cloves garlic, minced
- 1 tbsp. grated ginger
- 1 tbsp. sesame oil
- 1 tbsp. chopped green onions for garnish (optional)

Directions:

1. To prepare the glaze, combine soy sauce, rice vinegar, honey or maple syrup, chopped garlic, grated ginger, and sesame oil in a mixing bowl.

2. Preheat the grill for medium-high heat.

3. Brush the glaze on both sides of the tofu pieces.

4. Grill tofu slices for 3-4 minutes each side, or until grill marks show and the tofu is cooked through.

5. Transfer the grilled tofu to a serving plate.

6. Garnish with chopped green onions if desired.

7. Serve hot.

Nutrition Information (per serving):

- Calories: 150
- Total Fat: 8g
- Saturated Fat: 1g
- Cholesterol: 0mg

- Sodium: 400mg

- Total Carbohydrates: 11g

- Dietary Fiber: 1g

- Sugars: 6g

- Protein: 10g

Spinach and Mushroom Stuffed Chicken Breast

Prep Time: 15 minutes
Cook Time: 25 minutes
Servings: 4

Ingredients:

- 4 boneless, skinless chicken breasts

- 2 cups fresh spinach leaves

- 1 cup sliced mushrooms

- 1/2 cup shredded mozzarella cheese

- 2 cloves garlic, minced

- 1 tbsp. olive oil

- Salt and pepper to taste

Directions:

1. Preheat the oven to 375° Fahrenheit (190° Celsius). Lightly oil a baking dish.

2. In a pan, heat the olive oil over medium heat. Cook for approximately 1 minute, or until the garlic is aromatic.

3. Add fresh spinach leaves and sliced mushrooms to the skillet. Cook for 3-4 minutes, or until the spinach wilts and the mushrooms soften. Remove from heat and let it cool slightly.

4. Create a pocket in each chicken breast, taking care not to cut all the way through.

5. Fill each chicken breast with the cooked spinach-mushroom mixture. Sprinkle shredded mozzarella cheese on top.

6. Season the filled chicken breasts with salt and pepper.

7. Place the filled chicken breasts in the prepared baking dish.

8. Bake for 20-25 minutes, or until the chicken is cooked through.

9. Serve hot.

Nutrition Information (per serving):

- Calories: 250
- Total Fat: 9g
- Saturated Fat: 2.5g
- Cholesterol: 90mg
- Sodium: 200mg
- Total Carbohydrates: 4g
- Dietary Fiber: 1g
- Sugars: 1g
- Protein: 38g

Roasted Vegetable Quinoa Bowl

Prep Time: 15 minutes
Cook Time: 25 minutes
Servings: 4

Ingredients:

- 1 cup quinoa, rinsed
- 2 cups vegetable broth
- 2 cups mixed vegetables (such as bell peppers, zucchini, cherry tomatoes, red onion)
- 2 tbsp. olive oil
- Salt and pepper to taste
- 1/4 cup chopped fresh parsley
- 1/4 cup crumbled feta cheese (optional)
- Lemon wedges for serving

Directions:

1. Preheat the oven to 400 °F (200 °C). Line a baking sheet with parchment paper.

2. In a saucepan, mix the quinoa and vegetable broth. Bring to a boil, then lower to a low heat, cover, and simmer for 15-20 minutes, or until the quinoa is cooked and the liquid is absorbed.

3. Meanwhile, sprinkle the veggies with olive oil, salt, and pepper on the prepared baking sheet.

4. Roast veggies in a preheated oven for 15-20 minutes, turning halfway through, until soft and faintly caramelized.

5. Fluff cooked quinoa with a fork before dividing into serving dishes.

6. Top the quinoa with roasted veggies.

7. Garnish with chopped fresh parsley and crumbled feta cheese if preferred.

8. Serve with lemon wedges to squeeze over the bowl.

Nutrition Information (per serving):

- Calories: 300
- Total Fat: 12g
- Saturated Fat: 2g
- Cholesterol: 5mg
- Sodium: 300mg
- Total Carbohydrates: 40g
- Dietary Fiber: 7g
- Sugars: 4g
- Protein: 9g

Black Bean and Corn Tacos with Avocado Salsa

Prep Time: 15 minutes
Cook Time: 10 minutes
Servings: 4

Ingredients:

For Black Bean and Corn Filling:

- 1 can (15 oz) black beans, rinsed and drained
- 1 cup corn kernels (fresh, frozen, or canned)
- 1 tsp. ground cumin
- 1/2 tsp. chili powder
- Salt and pepper to taste

For Avocado Salsa:

- 1 ripe avocado, diced
- 1 tomato, diced
- 1/4 cup diced red onion
- 1/4 cup chopped fresh cilantro
- 1 tbsp. lime juice
- Salt and pepper to taste

For Tacos:

- 8 small whole wheat tortillas
- Additional toppings such as shredded lettuce, diced tomatoes, sliced jalapeños

Directions:

For Black Bean and Corn Filling:

1. In a pan, mix together black beans, corn kernels, ground cumin, chili powder, salt, and pepper. Cook over medium heat for 5-7 minutes, stirring periodically, until well cooked.

For Avocado Salsa:

1. In a mixing dish, add diced avocado, tomato, red onion, cilantro, lime juice, salt, and pepper. Gently toss to mix.

Assembling Tacos:

1. Warm the whole wheat tortillas according to the package directions.
2. Spoon the black bean and corn filling onto each tortilla.
3. Add avocado salsa, shredded lettuce, chopped tomatoes, and sliced jalapeños as desired.

4. Serve immediately.

Nutrition Information (per serving, including 2 tacos):

- Calories: 300

- Total Fat: 9g

- Saturated Fat: 1.5g

- Cholesterol: 0mg

- Sodium: 250mg

- Total Carbohydrates: 45g

- Dietary Fiber: 9g

- Sugars: 5g

- Protein: 12g

Broiled Cod with Tomato-Caper Relish

Prep Time: 10 minutes
Cook Time: 10 minutes
Servings: 4

Ingredients:

- 4 cod fillets

- 2 tbsp. olive oil

- Salt and pepper to taste

For Tomato-Caper Relish:

- 1 cup diced tomatoes

- 2 tbsp. capers, drained

- 1 tbsp. chopped fresh parsley

- 1 tbsp. lemon juice

- 1 tbsp. extra virgin olive oil

- Salt and pepper to taste

Directions:

1. Preheat the broiler.

2. Brush olive oil over fish fillets and season with salt and pepper.

3. Place the fish fillets on a broiler pan or baking sheet covered with aluminum foil.

4. Broil cod fillets for 4-5 minutes on each side, or until well done and readily flaked with a fork.

For Tomato-Caper Relish:

1. In a mixing dish, add diced tomatoes, capers, chopped fresh parsley, lemon juice, extra virgin olive oil, salt, and pepper.

2. Serve broiled fish fillets with tomato-caper relish spooned on top.

Nutrition Information (per serving):

- Calories: 200
- Total Fat: 9g
- Saturated Fat: 1.5g
- Cholesterol: 50mg
- Sodium: 250mg
- Total Carbohydrates: 5g
- Dietary Fiber: 1g
- Sugars: 2g
- Protein: 25g

Quinoa and Vegetable Salad

Prep Time: 15 minutes
Cook Time: 20 minutes
Servings: 4

Ingredients:

- 1 cup quinoa, rinsed
- 2 cups water or vegetable broth
- 1 cup diced cucumber
- 1 cup cherry tomatoes, halved
- 1 cup diced bell peppers (any color)
- 1/4 cup chopped fresh parsley
- 1/4 cup chopped fresh mint
- 2 tbsp. extra virgin olive oil
- 2 tbsp. lemon juice
- Salt and pepper to taste

Directions:

1. In a saucepan, mix the quinoa and water or vegetable broth. Bring to a boil, then decrease heat to low, cover, and cook for 15-20 minutes, or until quinoa is tender and liquid has been absorbed.

2. Fluff cooked quinoa with a fork and set aside to cool to room temperature.

3. In a large bowl, add cooked quinoa, diced cucumber, cherry tomatoes, diced bell peppers, parsley, and mint.

4. Make the dressing by whisking together extra virgin olive oil, lemon juice, salt, and pepper in a small bowl.

5. Pour the dressing over the quinoa and veggie mix. Toss until evenly coated.

6. Serve either cold or at room temperature.

Nutrition Information (per serving):

- Calories: 250

- Total Fat: 10g

- Saturated Fat: 1.5g

- Cholesterol: 0mg

- Sodium: 20mg

- Total Carbohydrates: 35g

- Dietary Fiber: 6g

- Sugars: 4g

- Protein: 7g

Roasted Garlic Cauliflower Mash

Prep Time: 10 minutes
Cook Time: 25 minutes
Servings: 4

Ingredients:

- 1 head cauliflower, cut into florets

- 2 tbsp. olive oil

- 4 cloves garlic, minced

- Salt and pepper to taste

- 1/4 cup low-fat milk (or unsweetened almond milk)

- 2 tbsp. chopped fresh chives (optional)

Directions:

1. Preheat the oven to 400 °F (200 °C). Line a baking sheet with parchment paper.

2. In a large mixing bowl, combine cauliflower florets, olive oil, minced garlic, salt, and pepper.

3. Spread the cauliflower mixture in a single layer on the prepared baking sheet.

4. Roast the cauliflower in a preheated oven for 20-25 minutes, or until soft and golden brown.

5. Transfer the roasted cauliflower to a food processor. Include low-fat milk.

6. Blend until smooth and creamy.

7. Season with more salt and pepper to taste.

8. If preferred, sprinkle with chopped fresh chives before serving.

Nutrition Information (per serving):

- Calories: 100

- Total Fat: 7g

- Saturated Fat: 1g

- Cholesterol: 0mg

- Sodium: 40mg

- Total Carbohydrates: 8g

- Dietary Fiber: 3g

- Sugars: 3g

- Protein: 3g

Steamed Broccoli with Lemon Garlic Sauce

Prep Time: 5 minutes
Cook Time: 10 minutes
Servings: 4

Ingredients:

- 1 lb broccoli florets

- 2 cloves garlic, minced

- 2 tbsp. olive oil

- 1 tbsp. lemon juice

- Salt and pepper to taste

- Lemon wedges for serving

Directions:

1. Steam broccoli florets for 5-7 minutes, or until tender.

2. Meanwhile, in a small pan, warm the olive oil over medium heat. Sauté minced garlic until fragrant, approximately 1 minute.

3. Remove skillet from heat and add lemon juice. Season with salt and pepper to taste.

4. Transfer the steamed broccoli to a serving dish. Drizzle with Lemon Garlic Sauce.

5. Serve hot, with lemon wedges to squeeze over the broccoli.

Nutrition Information (per serving):

- Calories: 90

- Total Fat: 7g

- Saturated Fat: 1g

- Cholesterol: 0mg

- Sodium: 30mg

- Total Carbohydrates: 6g

- Dietary Fiber: 3g

- Sugars: 2g

- Protein: 3g

Balsamic Glazed Brussels Sprouts

Prep Time: 10 minutes
Cook Time: 20 minutes
Servings: 4

Ingredients:

- 1 lb Brussels sprouts, trimmed and halved

- 2 tbsp. olive oil

- 2 tbsp. balsamic vinegar

- 1 tbsp. honey or maple syrup

- Salt and pepper to taste

Directions:

1. Preheat the oven to 400 °F (200 °C). Line a baking sheet with parchment paper.

2. In a mixing dish, combine Brussels sprouts, olive oil, balsamic vinegar, honey or maple syrup, salt, and pepper.

3. Spread the Brussels sprouts in a single layer on the prepared baking sheet.

4. Roast the Brussels sprouts in a warm oven for 20-25 minutes, or until tender and caramelized.

5. Serve hot.

Nutrition Information (per serving):

- Calories: 100
- Total Fat: 5g
- Saturated Fat: 1g
- Cholesterol: 0mg
- Sodium: 30mg
- Total Carbohydrates: 12g
- Dietary Fiber: 4g
- Sugars: 5g
- Protein: 4g

Spinach and Strawberry Salad

Prep Time: 10 minutes
Servings: 4

Ingredients:

- 6 cups fresh spinach leaves
- 1 cup sliced strawberries
- 1/4 cup crumbled feta cheese
- 1/4 cup sliced almonds
- 2 tbsp. balsamic vinegar

- 1 tbsp. extra virgin olive oil

- 1 tsp. honey or maple syrup

- Salt and pepper to taste

Directions:

1. In a large mixing dish, add fresh spinach leaves, sliced strawberries, crumbled feta cheese, and sliced almonds.

2. To create the dressing, combine the balsamic vinegar, extra virgin olive oil, honey or maple syrup, salt, and pepper in a small mixing bowl.

3. Pour the dressing over the salad and toss to coat evenly.

4. Serve immediately.

Nutrition Information (per serving):

- Calories: 150

- Total Fat: 10g

- Saturated Fat: 2g

- Cholesterol: 5mg

- Sodium: 150mg

- Total Carbohydrates: 13g

- Dietary Fiber: 4g

- Sugars: 6g

- Protein: 5g

Herb-Roasted Sweet Potatoes

Prep Time: 10 minutes
Cook Time: 30 minutes
Servings: 4

Ingredients:

- 2 large sweet potatoes, peeled and cut into cubes

- 2 tbsp. olive oil

- 1 tsp. dried thyme

- 1 tsp. dried rosemary

- 1 tsp. dried oregano

- Salt and pepper to taste

Directions:

1. Preheat the oven to 400 °F (200 °C). Line a baking sheet with parchment paper.

2. In a large mixing bowl, combine sweet potato cubes, olive oil, dried thyme, rosemary, oregano, salt, and pepper.

3. Place the sweet potato cubes in a single layer on the prepared baking sheet.

4. Roast the sweet potatoes in a preheated oven for 25-30 minutes, or until soft and golden brown.

5. Serve hot.

Nutrition Information (per serving):

- Calories: 150

- Total Fat: 7g

- Saturated Fat: 1g

- Cholesterol: 0mg

- Sodium: 60mg

- Total Carbohydrates: 21g

- Dietary Fiber: 4g

- Sugars: 6g

- Protein: 2g

Grilled Asparagus with Lemon Zest

Prep Time: 5 minutes
Cook Time: 10 minutes
Servings: 4

Ingredients:

- 1 lb asparagus spears, trimmed

- 2 tbsp. olive oil

- Zest of 1 lemon

- Salt and pepper to taste

- Lemon wedges for serving

Directions:

1. Preheat the grill for medium-high heat.

2. In a mixing bowl, combine asparagus spears, olive oil, lemon zest, salt, and pepper.

3. Grill asparagus spears for 3-4 minutes each side, or until tender and slightly browned.

4. Transfer the grilled asparagus to a serving plate.

5. Serve hot, with lemon wedges to squeeze over the asparagus.

Nutrition Information (per serving):

- Calories: 60

- Total Fat: 5g

- Saturated Fat: 1g

- Cholesterol: 0mg

- Sodium: 0mg

- Total Carbohydrates: 4g

- Dietary Fiber: 2g

- Sugars: 2g

- Protein: 2g

Lemon Herb Quinoa Pilaf

Prep Time: 10 minutes
Cook Time: 20 minutes
Servings: 4

Ingredients:

- 1 cup quinoa, rinsed

- 2 cups vegetable broth

- Zest of 1 lemon

- 2 tbsp. lemon juice

- 2 tbsp. chopped fresh parsley

- 1 tbsp. chopped fresh dill

- Salt and pepper to taste

Directions:

1. In a saucepan, mix the quinoa and vegetable broth. Bring to a boil, then lower to a low heat, cover, and simmer for 15-20 minutes, or until the quinoa is cooked and the liquid is absorbed.

2. Fluff cooked quinoa using a fork.

3. Mix in the lemon zest, lemon juice, chopped parsley, chopped dill, salt, and pepper.

4. Serve hot.

Nutrition Information (per serving):

- Calories: 180

- Total Fat: 3g

- Saturated Fat: 0g

- Cholesterol: 0mg

- Sodium: 400mg

- Total Carbohydrates: 32g

- Dietary Fiber: 4g

- Sugars: 1g

- Protein: 6g

Roasted Beet and Arugula Salad

Prep Time: 10 minutes
Cook Time: 45 minutes
Servings: 4

Ingredients:

- 4 medium beets, peeled and cut into cubes
- 2 tbsp. olive oil
- Salt and pepper to taste
- 4 cups arugula
- 1/4 cup crumbled goat cheese
- 2 tbsp. balsamic vinegar
- 1 tbsp. honey or maple syrup

Directions:

1. Preheat the oven to 400 °F (200 °C). Line a baking sheet with parchment paper.
2. In a mixing dish, combine beet cubes, olive oil, salt, and pepper.
3. Spread the beet cubes in a single layer on the prepared baking sheet.
4. Roast the beets in a warm oven for 40-45 minutes, or until soft and caramelized.
5. Let the cooked beets cool slightly.
6. In a large bowl, mix the arugula and roasted beet chunks.
7. To create the dressing, whisk together balsamic vinegar, honey, or maple syrup in a small mixing dish.
8. Drizzle the dressing over the salad and toss to distribute evenly.
9. Before serving, sprinkle the salad with crumbled goat cheese.

Nutrition Information (per serving):

- Calories: 150
- Total Fat: 9g
- Saturated Fat: 2g
- Cholesterol: 5mg

- Sodium: 150mg

- Total Carbohydrates: 15g

- Dietary Fiber: 4g

- Sugars: 10g

- Protein: 4g

Green Bean Almondine

Prep Time: 10 minutes
Cook Time: 10 minutes
Servings: 4

Ingredients:

- 1 lb green beans, trimmed

- 2 tbsp. olive oil

- 1/4 cup sliced almonds

- 2 cloves garlic, minced

- 1 tbsp. lemon juice

- Salt and pepper to taste

Directions:

1. Heat a big saucepan of water to a boil. Add the green beans and blanch for 2-3 minutes, or until tender-crisp. Drain and put aside.

2. In a pan, heat the olive oil over medium heat. Combine the sliced almonds and minced garlic. Sauté until the almonds are golden brown and aromatic, approximately 2-3 minutes.

3. Add the blanched green beans to the skillet. Drizzle with lemon juice.

4. Toss until uniformly coated with the almond-garlic mixture.

5. Season with salt and pepper to taste.

6. Serve hot.

Nutrition Information (per serving):

- Calories: 150

- Total Fat: 11g

- Saturated Fat: 1.5g

- Cholesterol: 0mg

- Sodium: 20mg

- Total Carbohydrates: 11g

- Dietary Fiber: 5g

- Sugars: 4g

- Protein: 5g

Cucumber Avocado Salad

Prep Time: 10 minutes
Servings: 4

Ingredients:

- 2 cucumbers, peeled and diced

- 1 avocado, diced

- 1/4 cup diced red onion

- 2 tbsp. chopped fresh cilantro

- 2 tbsp. lime juice

- 1 tbsp. extra virgin olive oil

- Salt and pepper to taste

Directions:

1. In a large mixing basin, add the diced cucumbers, avocado, red onion, and fresh cilantro.

2. The dressing is made by whisking together lime juice, extra virgin olive oil, salt, and pepper in a small bowl.

3. Pour the dressing over the salad and toss to coat evenly.

4. Serve immediately.

Nutrition Information (per serving):

- Calories: 150
- Total Fat: 11g
- Saturated Fat: 1.5g
- Cholesterol: 0mg
- Sodium: 20mg
- Total Carbohydrates: 14g
- Dietary Fiber: 6g
- Sugars: 4g
- Protein: 3g

Lemony Kale Salad with Avocado

Prep Time: 10 minutes
Cook Time: 0 minutes
Servings: 4

Ingredients:

- 1 bunch kale, stems removed and leaves thinly sliced

- 1 avocado, diced

- 1 lemon, juiced

- 2 tbsp. extra virgin olive oil

- Salt and pepper to taste

- Optional: toasted nuts or seeds for garnish

Directions:

1. Massage the kale in a large bowl with lemon juice and olive oil for 2-3 minutes, or until it softens slightly.

2. Add the cubed avocado to the bowl.

3. Season with salt and pepper to taste.

4. Toss gently until combined.

5. Garnish with roasted nuts or seeds if preferred.

6. Serve immediately.

Nutrition Information (per serving):

- Calories: 150

- Total Fat: 12g

- Saturated Fat: 2g

- Cholesterol: 0mg

- Sodium: 15mg

- Total Carbohydrates: 10g

- Dietary Fiber: 5g

- Sugars: 1g

- Protein: 3g

Mediterranean Quinoa Salad with Roasted Vegetables

Prep Time: 15 minutes
Cook Time: 25 minutes
Servings: 4

Ingredients:

- 1 cup quinoa, rinsed

- 2 cups water or vegetable broth

- 2 cups mixed vegetables (such as bell peppers, zucchini, cherry tomatoes, red onion), diced

- 2 tbsp. olive oil

- 1 tsp. dried oregano

- 1 tsp. dried basil

- 1/4 cup crumbled feta cheese

- Salt and pepper to taste

- Optional: lemon wedges for serving

Directions:

1. Preheat the oven to 400 °F (200 °C). Line a baking sheet with parchment paper.

2. In a saucepan, mix the quinoa with the water or vegetable broth. Bring to a boil, then lower to a low heat, cover, and simmer for 15-20 minutes, or until the quinoa is cooked and the liquid is absorbed.

3. Meanwhile, combine the veggies with olive oil, dried oregano, dried basil, salt, and pepper on the prepared baking sheet.

4. Roast veggies in a preheated oven for 20-25 minutes, turning halfway through, until soft and faintly caramelized.

5. In a large bowl, mix the cooked quinoa and roasted veggies.

6. Sprinkle crumbled feta cheese over the salad.

7. Serve warm or room temperature, with lemon wedges to squeeze over the salad.

Nutrition Information (per serving):

- Calories: 250

- Total Fat: 10g

- Saturated Fat: 2.5g

- Cholesterol: 5mg

- Sodium: 200mg

- Total Carbohydrates: 30g

- Dietary Fiber: 5g

- Sugars: 3g

- Protein: 8g

Citrus Beet and Arugula Salad

Prep Time: 15 minutes
Cook Time: 45 minutes (for roasting beets)
Servings: 4

Ingredients:

- 4 medium beets, trimmed and scrubbed

- 4 cups arugula

- 1 orange, peeled and segmented

- 1 grapefruit, peeled and segmented

- 1/4 cup crumbled goat cheese

- 2 tbsp. balsamic vinegar

- 1 tbsp. honey or maple syrup

- 2 tbsp. extra virgin olive oil

- Salt and pepper to taste

Directions:

1. Preheat the oven to 400 °F (200 °C). Wrap each beet in aluminum foil and set it on a baking pan.

2. Roast beets in a preheated oven for 40-45 minutes, or until fork-tender.

3. Let the roasted beets cool somewhat before peeling and dicing them.

4. In a large mixing bowl, add arugula, roasted beet cubes, orange, and grapefruit segments.

5. To prepare the dressing, mix together balsamic vinegar, honey or maple syrup, extra virgin olive oil, salt, and pepper in a small bowl.

6. Pour the dressing over the salad and toss to coat evenly.

7. Before serving, sprinkle the salad with crumbled goat cheese.

Nutrition Information (per serving):

- Calories: 200

- Total Fat: 9g

- Saturated Fat: 2g

- Cholesterol: 5mg

- Sodium: 150mg

- Total Carbohydrates: 27g

- Dietary Fiber: 6g

- Sugars: 19g

- Protein: 5g

Grilled Vegetable Platter with Balsamic Glaze

Prep Time: 15 minutes
Cook Time: 15 minutes
Servings: 4

Ingredients:

- Assorted vegetables (such as bell peppers, zucchini, eggplant, mushrooms, asparagus)
- 2 tbsp. olive oil
- Salt and pepper to taste
- Balsamic glaze for drizzling

Directions:

1. Preheat the grill for medium-high heat.
2. Cut the veggies into big pieces.
3. Toss the veggies with olive oil, salt, and pepper.
4. Grill veggies for 5-7 minutes each side, or until tender and slightly browned.
5. Arrange the grilled veggies on a dish.
6. Drizzle with balsamic glaze before serving.

Nutrition Information (per serving):

- Varies depending on vegetables used

Spinach and Strawberry Salad with Poppyseed Dressing

Prep Time: 10 minutes
Cook Time: 0 minutes
Servings: 4

Ingredients:

- 6 cups fresh spinach leaves
- 1 cup sliced strawberries
- 1/4 cup sliced almonds
- 2 tbsp. balsamic vinegar
- 1 tbsp. honey or maple syrup
- 1 tbsp. Dijon mustard
- 1/4 cup extra virgin olive oil
- 1 tbsp. poppy seeds

- Salt and pepper to taste

Directions:

1. In a large mixing dish, add fresh spinach leaves, sliced strawberries, and sliced almonds.

2. To prepare the dressing, combine balsamic vinegar, honey or maple syrup, Dijon mustard, extra virgin olive oil, poppy seeds, salt, and pepper in a small bowl.

3. Pour the dressing over the salad and toss to coat evenly.

4. Serve immediately.

Nutrition Information (per serving):

- Calories: 200

- Total Fat: 16g

- Saturated Fat: 2g

- Cholesterol: 0mg

- Sodium: 50mg

- Total Carbohydrates: 15g

- Dietary Fiber: 4g

- Sugars: 8g

- Protein: 4g

Roasted Cauliflower and Chickpea Salad

Prep Time: 10 minutes
Cook Time: 30 minutes
Servings: 4

Ingredients:

- 1 head cauliflower, cut into florets

- 1 can (15 oz) chickpeas, rinsed and drained

- 2 tbsp. olive oil

- 1 tsp. ground cumin

- 1 tsp. smoked paprika

- Salt and pepper to taste
- 4 cups mixed salad greens
- 1/4 cup tahini
- 2 tbsp. lemon juice
- 1 clove garlic, minced
- Water (as needed to thin the dressing)

Directions:

1. Preheat the oven to 400 °F (200 °C). Line a baking sheet with parchment paper.
2. In a large mixing bowl, combine cauliflower florets and chickpeas with olive oil, ground cumin, smoked paprika, salt, and pepper.
3. Place the cauliflower and chickpea mixture in a single layer on the prepared baking sheet.
4. Roast in the preheated oven for 25-30 minutes, or until the cauliflower is soft and the chickpeas are crunchy.
5. To prepare the dressing, mix together tahini, lemon juice, minced garlic, and water.
6. Arrange the mixed salad greens on serving dishes.
7. Top with the roasted cauliflower and chickpea mixture.
8. Drizzle with the tahini dressing before serving.

Nutrition Information (per serving):

- Calories: 300
- Total Fat: 18g
- Saturated Fat: 2.5g
- Cholesterol: 0mg
- Sodium: 350mg
- Total Carbohydrates: 28g
- Dietary Fiber: 9g
- Sugars: 5g
- Protein: 10g

Garden Fresh Tomato and Basil Salad

Prep Time: 10 minutes
Cook Time: 0 minutes
Servings: 4

Ingredients:

- 4 large tomatoes, sliced
- 1/4 cup fresh basil leaves, torn
- 2 tbsp. balsamic vinegar
- 1 tbsp. extra virgin olive oil
- Salt and pepper to taste
- Optional: crumbled feta cheese for garnish

Directions:

1. Arrange the tomato slices on a serving plate.
2. Sprinkle torn basil leaves over the tomato slices.
3. Drizzle balsamic vinegar and extra virgin olive oil over the salad.
4. Season with salt and pepper to taste.
5. If preferred, top the salad with crumbled feta cheese before serving.

Nutrition Information (per serving):

- Calories: 60
- Total Fat: 3g
- Saturated Fat: 0.5g
- Cholesterol: 0mg
- Sodium: 15mg
- Total Carbohydrates: 8g
- Dietary Fiber: 2g
- Sugars: 4g

- Protein: 2g

Asian-Inspired Edamame and Cabbage Slaw

Prep Time: 15 minutes
Cook Time: 0 minutes
Servings: 4

Ingredients:

- 2 cups shredded cabbage (green or purple)
- 1 cup shelled edamame, cooked according to package instructions
- 1 carrot, shredded
- 1/4 cup chopped fresh cilantro
- 2 tbsp. rice vinegar
- 1 tbsp. low-sodium soy sauce
- 1 tbsp. honey or maple syrup
- 1 tbsp. sesame oil
- 1 tsp. grated ginger
- 1 clove garlic, minced
- Salt and pepper to taste
- Optional: toasted sesame seeds for garnish

Directions:

1. In a large mixing dish, add shredded cabbage, cooked edamame, shredded carrot, and chopped cilantro.

2. To prepare the dressing, combine rice vinegar, low-sodium soy sauce, honey or maple syrup, sesame oil, grated ginger, chopped garlic, salt, and pepper in a small mixing bowl.

3. Pour the dressing over the cabbage mixture and toss to evenly coat.

4. If desired, top the slaw with toasted sesame seeds before serving.

Nutrition Information (per serving):

- Calories: 120

- Total Fat: 5g

- Saturated Fat: 0.5g

- Cholesterol: 0mg

- Sodium: 180mg

- Total Carbohydrates: 14g

- Dietary Fiber: 4g

- Sugars: 6g

- Protein: 7g

Roasted Sweet Potato and Brussels Sprouts Salad

Prep Time: 15 minutes
Cook Time: 30 minutes
Servings: 4

Ingredients:

- 2 sweet potatoes, peeled and diced

- 1 lb Brussels sprouts, trimmed and halved

- 2 tbsp. olive oil

- 1 tsp. smoked paprika

- 1 tsp. garlic powder

- Salt and pepper to taste

- 1/4 cup dried cranberries

- 1/4 cup chopped pecans

- 2 tbsp. balsamic glaze

Directions:

1. Preheat the oven to 400 °F (200 °C). Line a baking sheet with parchment paper.

2. In a large mixing bowl, combine diced sweet potatoes and half Brussels sprouts with olive oil, smoked paprika, garlic powder, salt, and pepper.

3. Place the sweet potatoes and Brussels sprouts in a single layer on the prepared baking sheet.

4. Roast in a preheated oven for 25-30 minutes, or until sweet potatoes are soft and Brussels sprouts have caramelized.

5. Transfer the roasted sweet potatoes and Brussels sprouts to a serving plate.

6. Sprinkle dried cranberries and chopped pecans over the salad.

7. Drizzle with balsamic glaze before serving.

Nutrition Information (per serving):

- Calories: 250

- Total Fat: 12g

- Saturated Fat: 1.5g

- Cholesterol: 0mg

- Sodium: 40mg

- Total Carbohydrates: 35g

- Dietary Fiber: 8g

- Sugars: 14g

- Protein: 5g

Greek Salad with Feta and Kalamata Olives

Prep Time: 15 minutes
Cook Time: 0 minutes
Servings: 4

Ingredients:

- 4 cups mixed salad greens

- 1 cucumber, diced

- 1 cup cherry tomatoes, halved

- 1/4 cup sliced red onion

- 1/4 cup crumbled feta cheese

- 1/4 cup pitted Kalamata olives

- 2 tbsp. extra virgin olive oil

- 2 tbsp. red wine vinegar

- 1 tsp. dried oregano

- Salt and pepper to taste

Directions:

1. In a large bowl, combine the mixed salad greens, diced cucumber, cherry tomatoes, sliced red onion, crumbled feta cheese, and pitted Kalamata olives.

2. The dressing is made by whisking together extra virgin olive oil, red wine vinegar, dried oregano, salt, and pepper in a small bowl.

3. Pour the dressing over the salad and toss to coat evenly.

4. Serve immediately.

Nutrition Information (per serving):

- Calories: 150

- Total Fat: 12g

- Saturated Fat: 2.5g

- Cholesterol: 10mg

- Sodium: 250mg

- Total Carbohydrates: 9g

- Dietary Fiber: 3g

- Sugars: 4g

- Protein: 3g

Summer Corn and Black Bean Salad

Prep Time: 15 minutes
Cook Time: 5 minutes
Servings: 4

Ingredients:

- 2 cups cooked corn kernels (fresh or thawed from frozen)

- 1 can (15 oz) black beans, rinsed and drained

- 1 red bell pepper, diced

- 1/4 cup chopped fresh cilantro

- 2 tbsp. lime juice

- 2 tbsp. extra virgin olive oil

- 1 tsp. ground cumin

- 1/2 tsp. chili powder

- Salt and pepper to taste

- Optional: diced avocado for serving

Directions:

1. In a large mixing dish, add cooked corn kernels, black beans, diced red bell pepper, and chopped fresh cilantro.

2. The dressing is made by whisking together lime juice, extra virgin olive oil, ground cumin, chili powder, salt, and pepper in a small bowl.

3. Pour the dressing over the salad and toss to coat evenly.

4. If preferred, garnish with cubed avocado before serving.

Nutrition Information (per serving):

- Calories: 200

- Total Fat: 7g

- Saturated Fat: 1g

- Cholesterol: 0mg

- Sodium: 150mg

- Total Carbohydrates: 30g

- Dietary Fiber: 8g

- Sugars: 3g

- Protein: 8g

Watermelon, Feta, and Mint Salad

Prep Time: 10 minutes
Cook Time: 0 minutes
Servings: 4

Ingredients:

- 4 cups cubed watermelon
- 1/2 cup crumbled feta cheese
- 2 tbsp. chopped fresh mint leaves
- 1 tbsp. balsamic glaze
- Optional: black pepper for garnish

Directions:

1. In a large mixing dish, add cubed watermelon, crumbled feta cheese, and chopped fresh mint leaves.
2. Drizzle the balsamic glaze over the salad.
3. Toss gently until combined.
4. If desired, season the salad with black pepper before serving.

Nutrition Information (per serving):

- Calories: 120
- Total Fat: 3g
- Saturated Fat: 2g
- Cholesterol: 15mg
- Sodium: 160mg
- Total Carbohydrates: 21g
- Dietary Fiber: 1g
- Sugars: 17g
- Protein: 4g

Grilled Salmon with Citrus Glaze

Prep Time: 10 minutes
Cook Time: 10 minutes
Servings: 4

Ingredients:

- 4 salmon fillets
- Salt and pepper to taste
- 1 tbsp. olive oil
- 1/4 cup orange juice
- 2 tbsp. lemon juice
- 2 tbsp. honey or maple syrup
- 1 tsp. grated ginger
- 1 clove garlic, minced
- 1 tbsp. chopped fresh parsley (for garnish)

Directions:

1. Preheat the grill for medium-high heat.
2. Season the salmon fillets with salt and pepper.
3. To prepare the glaze, combine olive oil, orange juice, lemon juice, honey or maple syrup, grated ginger, and chopped garlic in a small mixing bowl.
4. Grill salmon fillets for 4-5 minutes each side, or until they flake easily with a fork.
5. Brush the salmon fillets with the citrus glaze during the last few minutes of cooking.
6. Transfer the cooked fish to a serving plate.
7. Before serving, garnish with finely chopped fresh parsley.

Nutrition Information (per serving):

- Calories: 300

- Total Fat: 15g

- Saturated Fat: 2.5g

- Cholesterol: 75mg

- Sodium: 70mg

- Total Carbohydrates: 10g

- Dietary Fiber: 0g

- Sugars: 9g

- Protein: 30g

Herb-Crusted Turkey Breast

Prep Time: 15 minutes
Cook Time: 1 hour
Servings: 4

Ingredients:

- 1 turkey breast (about 2 lbs)

- 2 tbsp. olive oil

- 2 cloves garlic, minced

- 1 tbsp. chopped fresh rosemary

- 1 tbsp. chopped fresh thyme

- 1 tbsp. chopped fresh parsley

- Salt and pepper to taste

Directions:

1. Preheat the oven to 375° Fahrenheit (190° Celsius).

2. In a small mixing bowl, add olive oil, minced garlic, chopped fresh rosemary, chopped fresh thyme, chopped fresh parsley, salt, and pepper to form the herb combination.

3. Place the turkey breast on a roasting pan or baking dish.

4. Rub the herb mixture over the whole surface of the turkey breast.

5. Cook the turkey breast in the preheated oven for 50-60 minutes, or until the internal temperature reaches 165°F (74°C).

6. Let the turkey breast rest for 10 minutes before slicing.

7. Serve hot.

Nutrition Information (per serving):

- Calories: 250

- Total Fat: 8g

- Saturated Fat: 1.5g

- Cholesterol: 100mg

- Sodium: 100mg

- Total Carbohydrates: 0g

- Dietary Fiber: 0g

- Sugars: 0g

- Protein: 45g

Lemon Garlic Chicken Stir-Fry

Prep Time: 15 minutes
Cook Time: 15 minutes
Servings: 4

Ingredients:

- 1 lb boneless, skinless chicken breasts, sliced

- 2 tbsp. olive oil

- 4 cloves garlic, minced

- Zest and juice of 1 lemon

- 2 cups mixed vegetables (such as bell peppers, snap peas, carrots)

- Salt and pepper to taste

- Chopped fresh parsley (for garnish)

Directions:

1. Heat the olive oil in a large pan or wok over medium-high heat.

2. Add the minced garlic and lemon zest to the skillet. Sauté for 1-2 minutes, until aromatic.

3. Add the cut chicken breasts to the skillet. Cook for 5-6 minutes until the chicken is fully done.

4. Add the mixed veggies to the skillet. Cook for another 4-5 minutes, until the veggies are tender-crisp.

5. Squeeze lemon juice over the stir fry.

6. Season with salt and pepper to taste.

7. Before serving, garnish with finely chopped fresh parsley.

8. Serve hot with rice or noodles.

Nutrition Information (per serving):

- Calories: 250
- Total Fat: 10g
- Saturated Fat: 1.5g
- Cholesterol: 80mg
- Sodium: 80mg
- Total Carbohydrates: 8g
- Dietary Fiber: 2g
- Sugars: 2g
- Protein: 30g

Balsamic Glazed Pork Tenderloin

Prep Time: 10 minutes
Cook Time: 25 minutes
Servings: 4

Ingredients:

- 1 lb pork tenderloin

- Salt and pepper to taste
- 2 tbsp. olive oil
- 1/4 cup balsamic vinegar
- 2 tbsp. honey or maple syrup
- 2 cloves garlic, minced
- 1 tsp. chopped fresh rosemary

Directions:

1. Preheat the oven to 400 °F (200 °C).
2. Season the pork tenderloin with salt and pepper.
3. Heat olive oil in an ovenproof skillet over medium-high heat.
4. Sear the pork tenderloin on all sides until browned, approximately 2-3 minutes each side.
5. To prepare the glaze, mix together balsamic vinegar, honey or maple syrup, minced garlic, and freshly chopped rosemary in a small basin.
6. Brush the glaze over the cooked pork tenderloin.
7. Transfer the skillet to the preheated oven.
8. Roast pork tenderloin for 20-25 minutes, or until the internal temperature reaches 145°F (63°C).
9. Let the pork tenderloin rest for 5 minutes before slicing.
10. Serve hot.

Nutrition Information (per serving):

- Calories: 250
- Total Fat: 10g
- Saturated Fat: 2g
- Cholesterol: 75mg
- Sodium: 60mg
- Total Carbohydrates: 10g
- Dietary Fiber: 0g

- Sugars: 8g

- Protein: 30g

Roasted Garlic and Herb Lamb Chops

Prep Time: 10 minutes
Cook Time: 20 minutes
Servings: 4

Ingredients:

- 8 lamb loin chops

- Salt and pepper to taste

- 4 cloves garlic, minced

- 2 tbsp. chopped fresh rosemary

- 2 tbsp. chopped fresh thyme

- 2 tbsp. olive oil

- Lemon wedges (for serving)

Directions:

1. Preheat the oven to 400 °F (200 °C).

2. Season the lamb loin chops with salt and pepper.

3. Make the herb combination in a small bowl by combining minced garlic, chopped fresh rosemary, chopped fresh thyme, and olive oil.

4. Rub the herb mixture evenly over the lamb chops.

5. Preheat an ovenproof skillet to medium-high heat.

6. Sear the lamb chops on both sides until browned, approximately 2-3 minutes each side.

7. Transfer the skillet to the preheated oven.

8. Roast lamb chops for 10-12 minutes for medium-rare, or longer if you wish.

9. Let the lamb chops rest for 5 minutes before serving.

10. Serve hot, with lemon wedges.

Nutrition Information (per serving):

- Calories: 350

- Total Fat: 25g

- Saturated Fat: 10g

- Cholesterol: 95mg

- Sodium: 70mg

- Total Carbohydrates: 2g

- Dietary Fiber: 0g

- Sugars: 0g

- Protein: 30g

Turkey and Vegetable Skewers with Yogurt Sauce

Prep Time: 20 minutes
Cook Time: 10 minutes
Servings: 4

Ingredients:

- 1 lb turkey breast, cut into cubes

- 2 bell peppers, cut into chunks

- 1 red onion, cut into chunks

- 8 cherry tomatoes

- 8 wooden skewers, soaked in water for 30 minutes

- Salt and pepper to taste

- Olive oil for brushing

- 1 cup plain Greek yogurt

- 1 tbsp. lemon juice

- 1 clove garlic, minced

- 1 tbsp. chopped fresh dill

- Salt and pepper to taste

Directions:

1. Preheat the grill for medium-high heat.

2. Thread turkey cubes, bell pepper pieces, red onion chunks, and cherry tomatoes onto skewers.

3. Season the skewers with salt and pepper.

4. Brush the skewers with olive oil.

5. Grill the skewers for 4-5 minutes each side, or until the turkey is fully cooked and the veggies are soft.

6. To prepare the yogurt sauce, whisk together plain Greek yogurt, lemon juice, minced garlic, chopped fresh dill, salt, and pepper in a small mixing dish.

7. Serve the turkey and veggie skewers with yogurt sauce on the side. Preheat the grill for medium-high heat.

8. Thread turkey cubes, bell pepper pieces, red onion chunks, and cherry tomatoes onto skewers.

9. Season the skewers with salt and pepper.

10. Brush the skewers with olive oil.

11. Grill the skewers for 4-5 minutes each side, or until the turkey is fully cooked and the veggies are soft.

12. To prepare the yogurt sauce, whisk together plain Greek yogurt, lemon juice, minced garlic, chopped fresh dill, salt, and pepper in a small mixing dish.

13. Serve the turkey and veggie skewers with yogurt sauce on the side.

Nutrition Information (per serving):

- Calories: 300
- Total Fat: 5g
- Saturated Fat: 1g
- Cholesterol: 85mg
- Sodium: 150mg
- Total Carbohydrates: 10g
- Dietary Fiber: 2g

- Sugars: 6g

- Protein: 45g

Ginger Soy Glazed Beef Stir-Fry

Prep Time: 15 minutes
Cook Time: 15 minutes
Servings: 4

Ingredients:

- 1 lb beef sirloin, thinly sliced

- 2 tbsp. soy sauce

- 1 tbsp. honey or maple syrup

- 1 tbsp. rice vinegar

- 1 tsp. grated ginger

- 2 cloves garlic, minced

- 2 tbsp. olive oil

- 2 cups mixed vegetables (such as bell peppers, broccoli, snow peas)

- Salt and pepper to taste

- Sesame seeds (for garnish)

Directions:

1. To prepare the glaze, whisk together soy sauce, honey or maple syrup, rice vinegar, grated ginger, and chopped garlic in a mixing bowl.

2. Heat the olive oil in a large pan or wok over medium-high heat.

3. Add the meat slices to the skillet. Cook for 2-3 minutes, until golden.

4. Add the mixed veggies to the skillet. Cook for an another 3-4 minutes, or until the veggies are soft and crispy.

5. Pour the glaze over the steak and veggies in the pan. Stir until evenly coated.

6. Cook for a further 1-2 minutes, until the sauce thickens slightly.

7. Season with salt and pepper to taste.

8. Garnish with sesame seeds before serving.

9. Serve hot with rice or noodles.

Nutrition Information (per serving):

- Calories: 300

- Total Fat: 15g

- Saturated Fat: 3g

- Cholesterol: 60mg

- Sodium: 500mg

- Total Carbohydrates: 15g

- Dietary Fiber: 3g

- Sugars: 8g

- Protein: 25g

Mediterranean Style Grilled Chicken Breast

Prep Time: 10 minutes
Cook Time: 15 minutes
Servings: 4

Ingredients:

- 4 boneless, skinless chicken breasts

- Salt and pepper to taste

- 2 tbsp. olive oil

- 2 cloves garlic, minced

- 1 tsp. dried oregano

- 1 tsp. dried basil

- 1/2 tsp. paprika

- Zest and juice of 1 lemon

Directions:

1. Preheat the grill for medium-high heat.

2. Season the chicken breasts with salt and pepper.

3. To create the marinade, whisk together olive oil, minced garlic, dried oregano, dried basil, paprika, lemon zest, and lemon juice in a small bowl.

4. Rub the marinade all over the chicken breasts.

5. Grill chicken breasts for 6-7 minutes each side, or until well done and no longer pink in the middle.

6. Transfer the grilled chicken breasts to a serving plate.

7. Serve hot.

Nutrition Information (per serving):

- Calories: 200

- Total Fat: 10g

- Saturated Fat: 1.5g

- Cholesterol: 80mg

- Sodium: 70mg

- Total Carbohydrates: 1g

- Dietary Fiber: 0g

- Sugars: 0g

- Protein: 25g

Herb-Marinated Grilled Steak Salad

Prep Time: 15 minutes
Cook Time: 15 minutes
Servings: 4

Ingredients:

- 1 lb sirloin steak

- Salt and pepper to taste

- 2 tbsp. olive oil

- 2 cloves garlic, minced
- 1 tsp. dried thyme
- 1 tsp. dried rosemary
- 1 tsp. dried oregano
- 4 cups mixed salad greens
- 1 cup cherry tomatoes, halved
- 1/2 red onion, thinly sliced
- Balsamic vinaigrette (for serving)

Directions:

1. Season the sirloin steak with salt and pepper.
2. To create the marinade, whisk together olive oil, minced garlic, dried thyme, rosemary, and oregano in a small bowl.
3. Rub the marinade all over the meat.
4. Allow steak to marinate for at least 30 minutes, or up to 2 hours in the fridge.
5. Preheat the grill for medium-high heat.
6. Grill steak for 4-5 minutes each side, or until desired doneness.
7. Allow steak to rest for 5 minutes before slicing thinly across the grain.
8. In a large mixing bowl, combine mixed salad greens, cherry tomatoes, and thinly sliced red onion.
9. Spread the sliced steak over the salad.
10. Serve with the balsamic vinaigrette on the side.

Nutrition Information (per serving):

- Calories: 300
- Total Fat: 15g
- Saturated Fat: 4.5g
- Cholesterol: 75mg
- Sodium: 90mg

- Total Carbohydrates: 6g

- Dietary Fiber: 2g

- Sugars: 2g

- Protein: 35g

Citrus Herb Shrimp Skewers

Prep Time: 20 minutes
Cook Time: 6 minutes
Servings: 4

Ingredients:

- 1 lb large shrimp, peeled and deveined

- Salt and pepper to taste

- Zest and juice of 1 lemon

- Zest and juice of 1 orange

- 2 cloves garlic, minced

- 2 tbsp. chopped fresh parsley

- 2 tbsp. chopped fresh cilantro

- 2 tbsp. olive oil

- 8 wooden skewers, soaked in water for 30 minutes

Directions:

1. Season the shrimp with salt, pepper, lemon, and orange zest.

2. Make the marinade in a small bowl by combining lemon juice, orange juice, minced garlic, chopped fresh parsley, chopped fresh cilantro, and olive oil.

3. Toss the shrimp in the marinade to ensure they are uniformly coated.

4. Cover and chill for at least 15 minutes, or up to 30.

5. Preheat the grill for medium-high heat.

6. Thread the marinated shrimp onto skewers.

7. Grill shrimp skewers for 2-3 minutes each side, or until they are pink and opaque.

8. Serve hot.

Nutrition Information (per serving):

- Calories: 150

- Total Fat: 7g

- Saturated Fat: 1g

- Cholesterol: 150mg

- Sodium: 200mg

- Total Carbohydrates: 4g

- Dietary Fiber: 0g

- Sugars: 1g

- Protein: 20g

Teriyaki Turkey Meatballs

Prep Time: 15 minutes
Cook Time: 20 minutes
Servings: 4

Ingredients:

- 1 lb ground turkey

- 1/4 cup breadcrumbs

- 1 egg

- 2 cloves garlic, minced

- 2 green onions, chopped

- 2 tbsp. soy sauce

- 1 tbsp. honey or maple syrup

- 1 tsp. grated ginger

- 1 tsp. sesame oil

- Salt and pepper to taste

- Sesame seeds and chopped green onions (for garnish)

Directions:

1. Preheat the oven to 400 °F (200 °C). Line a baking sheet with parchment paper.

2. In a large mixing bowl, add ground turkey, breadcrumbs, egg, minced garlic, chopped green onions, soy sauce, honey or maple syrup, grated ginger, sesame oil, salt, and pepper. Mix until well mixed.

3. Form the mixture into meatballs and put on the prepared baking sheet.

4. Bake meatballs in a preheated oven for 18-20 minutes, or until well cooked and browned.

5. Remove the meatballs from the oven and allow them to cool slightly.

6. Before serving, garnish with sesame seeds and chopped green onions.

7. Serve hot with rice or noodles.

Nutrition Information (per serving):

- Calories: 250
- Total Fat: 10g
- Saturated Fat: 2g
- Cholesterol: 120mg
- Sodium: 400mg
- Total Carbohydrates: 10g
- Dietary Fiber: 1g
- Sugars: 4g
- Protein: 30g

Moroccan Spiced Chicken Tagine

Prep Time: 20 minutes
Cook Time: 40 minutes
Servings: 4

Ingredients:

- 4 bone-in, skinless chicken thighs
- Salt and pepper to taste
- 2 tbsp. olive oil
- 1 onion, finely chopped
- 2 cloves garlic, minced
- 1 tsp. ground cumin
- 1 tsp. ground coriander
- 1/2 tsp. ground cinnamon
- 1/2 tsp. ground ginger
- 1/4 tsp. ground turmeric
- Pinch of saffron threads
- 1 can (14 oz) diced tomatoes
- 1 cup chicken broth
- 1/4 cup chopped fresh cilantro
- 1/4 cup chopped fresh parsley
- Lemon wedges (for serving)

Directions:

1. Season the chicken thighs with salt and pepper.

2. Heat the olive oil in a tagine or large pan over medium heat.

3. Brown the chicken thighs on both sides for about 4-5 minutes each side. Remove and put aside.

4. In the same tagine or pan, combine the chopped onion and minced garlic. Sauté until softened, approximately 3-4 minutes.

5. Combine the ground cumin, ground coriander, ground cinnamon, ground ginger, ground turmeric, and saffron threads. Cook for 1-2 minutes, until aromatic.

6. Stir in the diced tomatoes and chicken broth.

7. Return the browned chicken thighs to the tagine or pan.

8. Cover and cook on low heat for 30 minutes, or until the chicken is tender.

9. Garnish with chopped fresh cilantro and parsley before serving.

10. Serve hot with lemon wedges, couscous, or rice.

Nutrition Information (per serving):

- Calories: 300
- Total Fat: 15g
- Saturated Fat: 3.5g
- Cholesterol: 100mg
- Sodium: 300mg
- Total Carbohydrates: 10g
- Dietary Fiber: 2g
- Sugars: 4g
- Protein: 30g

Grilled Lemon Garlic Salmon

Prep Time: 10 minutes
Cook Time: 10 minutes
Servings: 4

Ingredients:

- 4 salmon fillets
- Salt and pepper to taste
- 2 tbsp. olive oil
- Zest and juice of 1 lemon
- 4 cloves garlic, minced
- 2 tbsp. chopped fresh parsley

Directions:

1. Preheat the grill for medium-high heat.
2. Season the salmon fillets with salt and pepper.
3. In a small bowl, combine olive oil, lemon zest, lemon juice, minced garlic, and fresh parsley.
4. Brush the lemon-garlic mixture over the salmon fillets.
5. Grill salmon fillets for 4-5 minutes each side, or until they flake easily with a fork.
6. If preferred, garnish with more lemon wedges and serve hot.

Nutrition Information (per serving):

- Calories: 300
- Total Fat: 20g
- Saturated Fat: 4g
- Cholesterol: 80mg
- Sodium: 100mg

- Total Carbohydrates: 2g

- Dietary Fiber: 0g

- Sugars: 0g

- Protein: 30g

Baked Herb-Crusted Tilapia

Prep Time: 10 minutes
Cook Time: 15 minutes
Servings: 4

Ingredients:

- 4 tilapia fillets

- Salt and pepper to taste

- 2 tbsp. olive oil

- 1/2 cup breadcrumbs

- 1 tbsp. chopped fresh parsley

- 1 tbsp. chopped fresh thyme

- 1 tbsp. chopped fresh rosemary

- 1 clove garlic, minced

Directions:

1. Preheat the oven to 400 °F (200 °C). Line a baking sheet with parchment paper.

2. Season the tilapia fillets with salt and pepper.

3. To prepare the herb crust, mix olive oil, breadcrumbs, chopped fresh parsley, chopped fresh thyme, chopped fresh rosemary, and minced garlic.

4. Place the herb crust on top of each tilapia fillet.

5. Place the coated tilapia fillets on the prepared baking sheet.

6. Bake in a preheated oven for 12-15 minutes, or until the fish is fully cooked and the crust is golden brown.

7. Serve hot with lemon slices, if preferred.

Nutrition Information (per serving):

- Calories: 200
- Total Fat: 10g
- Saturated Fat: 2g
- Cholesterol: 60mg
- Sodium: 150mg
- Total Carbohydrates: 5g
- Dietary Fiber: 1g
- Sugars: 0g
- Protein: 25g

Seared Scallops with Citrus Salsa

Prep Time: 15 minutes
Cook Time: 5 minutes
Servings: 4

Ingredients:

- 16 large sea scallops
- Salt and pepper to taste
- 2 tbsp. olive oil
- Zest and juice of 1 lime
- Zest and juice of 1 orange
- 1 jalapeño, seeded and finely chopped
- 1/4 cup chopped fresh cilantro
- 1/4 cup chopped red onion

Directions:

1. Pat the scallops dry with paper towels and season with salt and pepper.
2. Heat olive oil in a large pan over medium-high heat.

3. Cook the scallops for 2-3 minutes on each side, or until golden brown and well cooked.

4. To prepare the citrus salsa, mix lime zest, lime juice, orange zest, orange juice, diced jalapeño, cilantro, and red onion.

5. Serve seared scallops hot, with citrus salsa spooned on top.

Nutrition Information (per serving):

- Calories: 150

- Total Fat: 5g

- Saturated Fat: 1g

- Cholesterol: 35mg

- Sodium: 350mg

- Total Carbohydrates: 5g

- Dietary Fiber: 1g

- Sugars: 2g

- Protein: 20g

Poached Halibut with Dill Sauce

Prep Time: 10 minutes
Cook Time: 10 minutes
Servings: 4

Ingredients:

- 4 halibut fillets

- Salt and pepper to taste

- 4 cups vegetable or fish broth

- Zest and juice of 1 lemon

- 1/4 cup chopped fresh dill

- 1/4 cup plain Greek yogurt

Directions:

1. Season the halibut fillets with salt and pepper.

2. In a large skillet or saucepan, bring vegetable or fish broth to a low simmer.

3. Carefully add the halibut fillets to the boiling stock.

4. Poach halibut fillets for 4-5 minutes, or until cooked through and opaque.

5. The dill sauce is made by whisking together lemon zest, lemon juice, chopped fresh dill, and plain Greek yogurt in a small bowl.

6. Serve poached halibut fillets hot, with dill sauce spooned on top.

Nutrition Information (per serving):

- Calories: 200

- Total Fat: 5g

- Saturated Fat: 1g

- Cholesterol: 40mg

- Sodium: 350mg

- Total Carbohydrates: 2g

- Dietary Fiber: 0g

- Sugars: 1g

- Protein: 35g

Cajun Shrimp and Quinoa Salad

Prep Time: 15 minutes
Cook Time: 15 minutes
Servings: 4

Ingredients:

- 1 cup quinoa

- 2 cups water or vegetable broth

- 1 lb large shrimp, peeled and deveined

- 2 tbsp. Cajun seasoning

- 2 tbsp. olive oil

- 1 red bell pepper, diced

- 1 yellow bell pepper, diced
- 1/2 red onion, diced
- 1/4 cup chopped fresh parsley
- 1/4 cup chopped fresh cilantro
- Zest and juice of 1 lime
- Salt and pepper to taste

Directions:

1. Rinse the quinoa under cool water. Heat water or vegetable broth in a pot until it boils. Add the quinoa, decrease the heat to low, cover, and simmer for 15 minutes, or until the quinoa is cooked and the liquid is absorbed. Remove from the heat and let it settle for 5 minutes, covered. Fluff with a fork and let to cool.

2. In a mixing dish, combine the shrimp and Cajun spice until evenly covered.

3. In a pan, heat olive oil over medium-high heat. Add the shrimp and cook for 2-3 minutes each side, or until pink and opaque. Remove from heat and let it cool slightly.

4. In a large mixing bowl, add the cooked quinoa, cooked shrimp, diced red and yellow bell peppers, diced red onion, chopped fresh parsley, chopped fresh cilantro, and lime zest and juice. Toss until evenly blended.

5. Season with salt and pepper to taste.

6. Serve the shrimp and quinoa salad refrigerated or at room temperature.

Nutrition Information (per serving):

- Calories: 300
- Total Fat: 10g
- Saturated Fat: 1.5g
- Cholesterol: 150mg
- Sodium: 500mg
- Total Carbohydrates: 30g
- Dietary Fiber: 5g
- Sugars: 3g
- Protein: 25g

Lemon Pepper Mahi Mahi

Prep Time: 10 minutes
Cook Time: 10 minutes
Servings: 4

Ingredients:

- 4 mahi mahi fillets

- Salt and pepper to taste

- 2 tbsp. olive oil

- Zest and juice of 1 lemon

- 1 tbsp. cracked black pepper

- 1 tbsp. chopped fresh parsley

Directions:

1. Season the mahi mahi fillets with salt and pepper.

2. In a small mixing bowl, add olive oil, lemon zest, lemon juice, crushed black pepper, and chopped fresh parsley.

3. Rub the lemon pepper mixture on the mahi mahi fillets.

4. Cook in a skillet over medium-high heat. Cook mahi mahi fillets for 4-5 minutes on each side, or until the fish is cooked through and readily flaked with a fork.

5. If preferred, garnish with more lemon wedges and serve hot.

Nutrition Information (per serving):

- Calories: 200

- Total Fat: 10g

- Saturated Fat: 2g

- Cholesterol: 80mg

- Sodium: 100mg

- Total Carbohydrates: 0g

- Dietary Fiber: 0g

- Sugars: 0g

- Protein: 25g

Teriyaki Glazed Cod

Prep Time: 10 minutes
Cook Time: 15 minutes
Servings: 4

Ingredients:

- 4 cod fillets

- Salt and pepper to taste

- 1/4 cup soy sauce

- 2 tbsp. honey or maple syrup

- 2 tbsp. rice vinegar

- 1 clove garlic, minced

- 1 tsp. grated ginger

- 1 tbsp. cornstarch

- 2 tbsp. water

- Sesame seeds (for garnish)

- Chopped green onions (for garnish)

Directions:

1. Preheat the oven to 400 °F (200 °C). Line a baking sheet with parchment paper.

2. Season cod fillets with salt and pepper before placing them on the prepared baking sheet.

3. In a small saucepan, mix together the soy sauce, honey or maple syrup, rice vinegar, chopped garlic, and grated ginger. Bring to a simmer over medium heat.

4. In a small bowl, combine cornstarch and water to form a slurry. Stir the slurry into the boiling sauce until it thickens.

5. Brush the teriyaki glaze on the fish fillets.

6. Bake in the preheated oven for 12-15 minutes, or until the fish is cooked through and readily flaked with a fork.

7. Before serving, garnish with sesame seeds and chopped green onions.

Nutrition Information (per serving):

- Calories: 200

- Total Fat: 2g

- Saturated Fat: 0g

- Cholesterol: 60mg

- Sodium: 600mg

- Total Carbohydrates: 15g

- Dietary Fiber: 0g

- Sugars: 10g

- Protein: 30g

Mediterranean-style Grilled Swordfish

Prep Time: 15 minutes
Cook Time: 10 minutes
Servings: 4

Ingredients:

- 4 swordfish steaks

- Salt and pepper to taste

- 2 tbsp. olive oil

- Zest and juice of 1 lemon

- 2 cloves garlic, minced

- 1 tsp. dried oregano

- 1 tsp. dried thyme

- 1 tsp. dried basil

Directions:

1. Season the swordfish steaks with salt and pepper.

2. To create the marinade, whisk together olive oil, lemon zest, lemon juice, minced garlic, dried oregano, dried thyme, and dried basil.

3. Rub the marinade evenly over the swordfish steaks.

4. Allow swordfish steaks to marinade for at least 30 minutes, or up to 2 hours, in the refrigerator.

5. Preheat the grill for medium-high heat.

6. Grill swordfish steaks for 4-5 minutes each side, or until the fish is cooked through and readily flaked with a fork.

7. If preferred, garnish with more lemon wedges and serve hot.

Nutrition Information (per serving):

- Calories: 250

- Total Fat: 12g

- Saturated Fat: 2g

- Cholesterol: 80mg

- Sodium: 300mg

- Total Carbohydrates: 2g

- Dietary Fiber: 0g

- Sugars: 0g

- Protein: 30g

Coconut Curry Shrimp Soup

Prep Time: 10 minutes
Cook Time: 20 minutes
Servings: 4

Ingredients:

- 1 tbsp. coconut oil

- 1 onion, diced

- 2 cloves garlic, minced
- 1 tbsp. grated ginger
- 2 tbsp. red curry paste
- 4 cups vegetable or chicken broth
- 1 can (14 oz) coconut milk
- 1 lb large shrimp, peeled and deveined
- 2 cups chopped mixed vegetables (such as bell peppers, carrots, broccoli)
- 2 tbsp. fish sauce (optional)
- Juice of 1 lime
- Chopped fresh cilantro (for garnish)

Directions:

1. In a large saucepan, melt coconut oil over medium heat.
2. Add the chopped onion, minced garlic, and grated ginger to the saucepan. Sauté until softened, approximately 3-4 minutes.
3. Stir in the red curry paste and simmer for 1-2 minutes, until aromatic.
4. Pour in the vegetable or chicken broth and coconut milk. Bring to a simmer.
5. Add the shrimp and mixed veggies to the saucepan. Cook for 5-7 minutes, or until the shrimp become pink and opaque and the veggies are soft.
6. Mix in the fish sauce (if using) and lime juice.
7. Pour the soup into bowls and top with chopped fresh cilantro before serving.

Nutrition Information (per serving):

- Calories: 300
- Total Fat: 20g
- Saturated Fat: 15g
- Cholesterol: 150mg
- Sodium: 700mg
- Total Carbohydrates: 10g

- Dietary Fiber: 2g

- Sugars: 3g

- Protein: 20g

Oven-Baked Lemon Herb Cod

Prep Time: 10 minutes
Cook Time: 15 minutes
Servings: 4

Ingredients:

- 4 cod fillets

- Salt and pepper to taste

- 2 tbsp. olive oil

- Zest and juice of 1 lemon

- 1 tbsp. chopped fresh parsley

- 1 tbsp. chopped fresh dill

- 1 clove garlic, minced

Directions:

1. Preheat the oven to 400 °F (200 °C). Line a baking sheet with parchment paper.

2. Season cod fillets with salt and pepper before placing them on the prepared baking sheet.

3. Make the herb combination in a small bowl by combining olive oil, lemon zest, lemon juice, chopped fresh parsley, chopped fresh dill, and minced garlic.

4. Brush the herb mixture on the fish fillets.

5. Bake in the preheated oven for 12-15 minutes, or until the fish is cooked through and readily flaked with a fork.

6. If preferred, garnish with more lemon wedges and serve hot.

Nutrition Information (per serving):

- Calories: 200

- Total Fat: 10g

- Saturated Fat: 1.5g

- Cholesterol: 60mg

- Sodium: 100mg

- Total Carbohydrates: 0g

- Dietary Fiber: 0g

- Sugars: 0g

- Protein: 25g

Spicy Sriracha Tuna Lettuce Wraps

Prep Time: 15 minutes
Cook Time: 5 minutes
Servings: 4

Ingredients:

- 2 cans (5 oz each) tuna, drained

- 2 tbsp. mayonnaise or Greek yogurt

- 1 tbsp. Sriracha sauce (adjust to taste)

- 1 tbsp. lime juice

- 1/4 cup diced red bell pepper

- 1/4 cup diced cucumber

- 2 green onions, thinly sliced

- Salt and pepper to taste

- 8 large lettuce leaves

Directions:

1. In a bowl, add the drained tuna, mayonnaise or Greek yogurt, Sriracha sauce, lime juice, chopped red bell pepper, diced cucumber, and thinly sliced green onions. Mix until well mixed.

2. Season with salt and pepper to taste.

3. Spoon the tuna mixture onto lettuce leaves.

4. Serve the hot Sriracha tuna lettuce wraps immediately.

Nutrition Information (per serving):

- Calories: 150

- Total Fat: 5g

- Saturated Fat: 1g

- Cholesterol: 30mg

- Sodium: 300mg

- Total Carbohydrates: 4g

- Dietary Fiber: 1g

- Sugars: 2g

- Protein: 20g

Grilled Shrimp and Vegetable Skewers

Prep Time: 20 minutes
Cook Time: 10 minutes
Servings: 4

Ingredients:

- 1 lb large shrimp, peeled and deveined

- 2 bell peppers, cut into chunks

- 1 red onion, cut into chunks

- 8 cherry tomatoes

- 8 wooden skewers, soaked in water for 30 minutes

- Salt and pepper to taste

- Olive oil for brushing

- Lemon wedges (for serving)

Directions:

1. Preheat the grill for medium-high heat.

2. Thread skewers with shrimp, bell pepper, red onion, and cherry tomatoes.

3. Season the skewers with salt and pepper.

4. Brush the skewers with olive oil.

5. Grill the skewers for 2-3 minutes each side, or until the shrimp are pink and opaque, and the veggies are soft.

6. Serve the grilled shrimp and veggie skewers hot with lemon wedges.

Nutrition Information (per serving):

- Calories: 150
- Total Fat: 5g
- Saturated Fat: 1g
- Cholesterol: 150mg
- Sodium: 200mg
- Total Carbohydrates: 5g
- Dietary Fiber: 1g
- Sugars: 2g
- Protein: 20g

Lentil and Vegetable Soup

Prep Time: 15 minutes
Cook Time: 45 minutes
Servings: 6

Ingredients:

- 1 cup dried green lentils, rinsed

- 6 cups vegetable broth

- 1 onion, diced

- 2 carrots, diced

- 2 celery stalks, diced

- 2 cloves garlic, minced

- 1 tsp. ground cumin

- 1 tsp. ground coriander

- 1/2 tsp. smoked paprika

- Salt and pepper to taste

- 2 cups chopped spinach or kale

- Juice of 1 lemon

- Chopped fresh parsley for garnish

Directions:

1. In a large saucepan, mix the lentils and the vegetable broth. Bring to a boil, then decrease heat to low and let simmer for 20 minutes.

2. Add the chopped onion, carrots, celery, minced garlic, ground cumin, ground coriander, smoked paprika, salt, and pepper to the saucepan. Simmer for another 20-25 minutes, or until the veggies are soft and the lentils are well cooked.

3. Mix in the chopped spinach or kale and lemon juice. Cook for a further five minutes.

4. Taste and adjust the seasoning as required.

5. Serve hot and garnish with chopped fresh parsley.

Nutrition Information (per serving):

- Calories: 200
- Total Fat: 1g
- Saturated Fat: 0g
- Cholesterol: 0mg
- Sodium: 700mg
- Total Carbohydrates: 38g
- Dietary Fiber: 16g
- Sugars: 5g
- Protein: 13g

Quinoa and Kale Stew

Prep Time: 15 minutes
Cook Time: 30 minutes
Servings: 6

Ingredients:

- 1 cup quinoa, rinsed
- 4 cups vegetable broth
- 1 onion, diced
- 2 carrots, diced
- 2 celery stalks, diced
- 2 cloves garlic, minced
- 1 tsp. dried thyme
- 1 tsp. dried rosemary
- 1 bay leaf
- Salt and pepper to taste

- 4 cups chopped kale

- Juice of 1 lemon

- Chopped fresh parsley for garnish

Directions:

1. In a large saucepan, mix the quinoa and vegetable broth. Bring to a boil, then decrease heat to low and let simmer for 15 minutes.

2. Add the chopped onion, carrots, celery, minced garlic, dried thyme, dried rosemary, bay leaf, salt, and pepper to the saucepan. Simmer for another 10-15 minutes, until the veggies are soft.

3. Stir in the chopped kale and lemon juice. Cook for another 5 minutes, or until the kale has wilted.

4. Remove the bay leaf before serving.

5. Serve hot and garnish with chopped fresh parsley.

Nutrition Information (per serving):

- Calories: 200

- Total Fat: 2g

- Saturated Fat: 0g

- Cholesterol: 0mg

- Sodium: 700mg

- Total Carbohydrates: 38g

- Dietary Fiber: 6g

- Sugars: 4g

- Protein: 9g

Turkey Chili with Beans

Prep Time: 15 minutes
Cook Time: 1 hour
Servings: 6

Ingredients:

- 1 tbsp. olive oil

- 1 onion, diced

- 2 cloves garlic, minced

- 1 lb ground turkey

- 2 tbsp. chili powder

- 1 tsp. ground cumin

- 1 tsp. dried oregano

- 1/2 tsp. paprika

- 1/4 tsp. cayenne pepper (optional)

- 1 can (14 oz) diced tomatoes

- 1 can (14 oz) kidney beans, drained and rinsed

- 1 can (14 oz) black beans, drained and rinsed

- 2 cups vegetable broth

- Salt and pepper to taste

- Chopped fresh cilantro for garnish

- Greek yogurt or sour cream for serving (optional)

Directions:

1. In a large saucepan, heat the olive oil over medium heat. Cook until the onion and garlic are softened, which should take around 5 minutes.

2. Cook the ground turkey, breaking it up with a spoon, until it is browned, approximately 5-7 minutes.

3. Cook for 1-2 minutes, stirring in the chili powder, powdered cumin, dried oregano, paprika, and cayenne pepper (if using), until aromatic.

4. Add the chopped tomatoes (with juices), kidney beans, black beans, and vegetable broth to the saucepan. Bring to a simmer.

5. Reduce the heat to low and cook uncovered for 45 minutes to an hour, stirring regularly, until the chili thickens and the flavors blend.

6. Season with salt and pepper to taste.

7. Serve hot, topped with chopped fresh cilantro and a dollop of Greek yogurt or sour cream if preferred.

Nutrition Information (per serving):

- Calories: 300

- Total Fat: 10g

- Saturated Fat: 2g

- Cholesterol: 50mg

- Sodium: 600mg

- Total Carbohydrates: 30g

- Dietary Fiber: 10g

- Sugars: 5g

- Protein: 25g

Butternut Squash Soup with Ginger

Prep Time: 15 minutes
Cook Time: 40 minutes
Servings: 6

Ingredients:

- 1 tbsp. olive oil

- 1 onion, diced

- 2 cloves garlic, minced

- 1 tbsp. grated ginger

- 1 butternut squash, peeled, seeded, and diced

- 4 cups vegetable broth

- 1 tsp. ground cumin

- 1/2 tsp. ground cinnamon

- 1/4 tsp. ground nutmeg

- Salt and pepper to taste

- Coconut milk for garnish (optional)

- Chopped fresh cilantro for garnish (optional)

Directions:

1. Heat olive oil in a large pot over medium heat. Add diced onion and minced garlic, and cook until softened, about 5 minutes.

2. Add grated ginger and diced butternut squash to the pot, and cook for an additional 5 minutes.

3. Stir in vegetable broth, ground cumin, ground cinnamon, and ground nutmeg. Bring to a boil, then reduce heat to low and simmer for 20-25 minutes, or until butternut squash is tender.

4. Using an immersion blender, puree the soup until smooth. Alternatively, transfer the soup to a blender and puree in batches until smooth, then return to the pot.

5. Season with salt and pepper to taste.

6. Serve hot, garnished with a swirl of coconut milk and chopped fresh cilantro if desired.

Nutrition Information (per serving):

- Calories: 150

- Total Fat: 3g

- Saturated Fat: 0.5g

- Cholesterol: 0mg

- Sodium: 600mg

- Total Carbohydrates: 30g

- Dietary Fiber: 5g

- Sugars: 5g

- Protein: 3g

Minestrone Soup with Whole Grain Pasta

Prep Time: 15 minutes
Cook Time: 30 minutes
Servings: 6

Ingredients:

- 1 tbsp. olive oil
- 1 onion, diced
- 2 carrots, diced
- 2 celery stalks, diced
- 2 cloves garlic, minced
- 1 can (14 oz) diced tomatoes
- 6 cups vegetable broth
- 1 tsp. dried oregano
- 1 tsp. dried basil
- 1/2 tsp. dried thyme
- 1/2 tsp. dried rosemary
- Salt and pepper to taste
- 1 cup whole grain pasta (such as penne or fusilli)
- 2 cups chopped spinach or kale
- Grated Parmesan cheese for garnish (optional)

Directions:

1. In a large saucepan, heat the olive oil over medium heat. Cook for 5 minutes, stirring in the chopped onion, carrots, celery, and minced garlic.

2. Mix in the chopped tomatoes (with liquids), vegetable broth, dried oregano, basil, thyme, and rosemary. Bring to a boil, then decrease heat to low and let simmer for 15 minutes.

3. Cook the whole grain pasta until al dente, following the package directions.

4. Add the chopped spinach or kale and simmer for another 2-3 minutes, or until wilted.

5. Season with salt and pepper to taste.

6. Serve hot, topped with grated Parmesan cheese if preferred.

Nutrition Information (per serving):

- Calories: 200

- Total Fat: 3g

- Saturated Fat: 0.5g

- Cholesterol: 0mg

- Sodium: 700mg

- Total Carbohydrates: 35g

- Dietary Fiber: 8g

- Sugars: 7g

- Protein: 7g

Spinach and White Bean Stew

Prep Time: 10 minutes
Cook Time: 30 minutes
Servings: 4

Ingredients:

- 1 tbsp. olive oil

- 1 onion, diced

- 2 cloves garlic, minced

- 1 tsp. dried Italian seasoning

- 1/4 tsp. red pepper flakes

- 1 can (14 oz) diced tomatoes

- 2 cups vegetable broth

- 2 cans (14 oz each) white beans (such as cannellini or Great Northern), drained and rinsed

- 4 cups chopped fresh spinach

- Salt and pepper to taste

- Grated Parmesan cheese for garnish (optional)

Directions:

1. In a large saucepan, heat the olive oil over medium heat. Cook until the onion and garlic are softened, which should take around 5 minutes.

2. Cook for a further 1-2 minutes, stirring in the dry Italian seasoning and red pepper flakes until aromatic.

3. Add the chopped tomatoes (with juices), vegetable broth, and white beans to the saucepan. Bring to a boil, then decrease heat to low and let simmer for 15 minutes.

4. Add the chopped fresh spinach and simmer for another 5 minutes, or until wilted.

5. Season with salt and pepper to taste.

6. Serve hot, topped with grated Parmesan cheese if preferred.

Nutrition Information (per serving):

- Calories: 250
- Total Fat: 3g
- Saturated Fat: 0.5g
- Cholesterol: 0mg
- Sodium: 800mg
- Total Carbohydrates: 45g
- Dietary Fiber: 12g
- Sugars: 4g
- Protein: 15g

Chicken and Vegetable Soup with Barley

Prep Time: 15 minutes
Cook Time: 1 hour
Servings: 6

Ingredients:

- 1 tbsp. olive oil
- 1 onion, diced
- 2 carrots, diced

- 2 celery stalks, diced

- 2 cloves garlic, minced

- 1 lb boneless, skinless chicken breasts, cut into bite-sized pieces

- 1/2 cup pearl barley

- 6 cups chicken broth

- 1 tsp. dried thyme

- 1 tsp. dried rosemary

- Salt and pepper to taste

- 2 cups chopped spinach or kale

- Chopped fresh parsley for garnish

Directions:

1. In a large saucepan, heat the olive oil over medium heat. Cook for 5 minutes, stirring in the chopped onion, carrots, celery, and minced garlic.

2. Cook the bite-sized chicken pieces in the saucepan for 5 minutes, or until browned.

3. Stir in the pearl barley, chicken broth, dried thyme, and rosemary. Bring to a boil, then lower to a low heat and simmer for 45 minutes to an hour, or until the barley is soft.

4. Stir in the chopped spinach or kale and simmer for another 5 minutes, or until wilted.

5. Season with salt and pepper to taste.

6. Serve hot and garnish with chopped fresh parsley.

Nutrition Information (per serving):

- Calories: 300

- Total Fat: 5g

- Saturated Fat: 1g

- Cholesterol: 50mg

- Sodium: 700mg

- Total Carbohydrates: 30g

- Dietary Fiber: 6g

- Sugars: 5g

- Protein: 30g

Moroccan Chickpea Stew

Prep Time: 15 minutes
Cook Time: 45 minutes
Servings: 6

Ingredients:

- 1 tbsp. olive oil

- 1 onion, diced

- 2 cloves garlic, minced

- 1 tbsp. grated ginger

- 1 tsp. ground cumin

- 1 tsp. ground coriander

- 1/2 tsp. ground cinnamon

- 1/4 tsp. cayenne pepper (optional)

- 2 cans (14 oz each) diced tomatoes

- 4 cups vegetable broth

- 2 cans (14 oz each) chickpeas (garbanzo beans), drained and rinsed

- 2 cups chopped carrots

- 2 cups chopped sweet potatoes

- Salt and pepper to taste

- Chopped fresh cilantro for garnish

Directions:

1. In a large saucepan, heat the olive oil over medium heat. Cook for approximately 5 minutes, or until the chopped onion has softened.

2. Cook for a further 1-2 minutes, stirring in minced garlic, grated ginger, ground cumin, ground coriander, ground cinnamon, and cayenne pepper (if using).

3. Add diced tomatoes (with juices), vegetable broth, chickpeas, sliced carrots, and chopped sweet potatoes. Bring to a boil, then lower to a low heat and cook for 30-40 minutes, or until veggies are soft.

4. Season with salt and pepper to taste.

5. Serve hot and garnish with chopped fresh cilantro.

Nutrition Information (per serving):

- Calories: 250

- Total Fat: 3g

- Saturated Fat: 0.5g

- Cholesterol: 0mg

- Sodium: 800mg

- Total Carbohydrates: 45g

- Dietary Fiber: 10g

- Sugars: 10g

- Protein: 10g

Tomato Basil Soup with Cannellini Beans

Prep Time: 10 minutes
Cook Time: 30 minutes
Servings: 6

Ingredients:

- 1 tbsp. olive oil

- 1 onion, diced

- 2 cloves garlic, minced

- 2 cans (14 oz each) diced tomatoes

- 4 cups vegetable broth

- 1 tsp. dried basil

- 1/2 tsp. dried oregano

- Salt and pepper to taste

- 2 cans (14 oz each) cannellini beans, drained and rinsed

- Chopped fresh basil for garnish

- Grated Parmesan cheese for garnish (optional)

Directions:

1. In a large saucepan, heat the olive oil over medium heat. Cook for approximately 5 minutes, or until the chopped onion has softened.

2. Add the minced garlic and simmer for another 1-2 minutes, or until fragrant.

3. Mix in the chopped tomatoes (with liquids), vegetable broth, dried basil, dry oregano, salt, and pepper. Bring to a boil, then decrease heat to low and let simmer for 20-25 minutes.

4. Using an immersion blender, purée the soup until smooth. Alternatively, put the soup to a blender and purée in stages until smooth before returning to the pot.

5. Stir in the cannellini beans and simmer for another 5 minutes.

6. Serve hot, topped with chopped fresh basil and grated Parmesan cheese if preferred.

Nutrition Information (per serving):

- Calories: 200

- Total Fat: 2g

- Saturated Fat: 0.5g

- Cholesterol: 0mg

- Sodium: 700mg

- Total Carbohydrates: 35g

- Dietary Fiber: 10g

- Sugars: 5g

- Protein: 10g

Cabbage and Potato Soup

Prep Time: 15 minutes
Cook Time: 40 minutes
Servings: 6

Ingredients:

- 1 tbsp. olive oil
- 1 onion, diced
- 2 cloves garlic, minced
- 4 cups shredded cabbage
- 2 large potatoes, peeled and diced
- 6 cups vegetable broth
- 1 tsp. dried thyme
- Salt and pepper to taste
- Chopped fresh parsley for garnish

Directions:

1. In a large saucepan, heat the olive oil over medium heat. Cook for approximately 5 minutes, or until the chopped onion has softened.
2. Add the minced garlic and simmer for another 1-2 minutes, or until fragrant.
3. Stir in the shredded cabbage and cubed potatoes, and simmer for 5 minutes.
4. Add the veggie stock and dried thyme to the saucepan. Bring to a boil, then decrease heat to low and let simmer for 30 minutes, or until potatoes are cooked.
5. Season with salt and pepper to taste.
6. Serve hot and garnish with chopped fresh parsley.

Nutrition Information (per serving):

- Calories: 150
- Total Fat: 3g
- Saturated Fat: 0.5g
- Cholesterol: 0mg

- Sodium: 700mg

- Total Carbohydrates: 30g

- Dietary Fiber: 6g

- Sugars: 5g

- Protein: 3g

Black Bean and Sweet Potato Chili

Prep Time: 15 minutes
Cook Time: 1 hour
Servings: 6

Ingredients:

- 1 tbsp. olive oil

- 1 onion, diced

- 2 cloves garlic, minced

- 2 sweet potatoes, peeled and diced

- 2 tsp. chili powder

- 1 tsp. ground cumin

- 1/2 tsp. smoked paprika

- 1/4 tsp. cayenne pepper (optional)

- 1 can (14 oz) diced tomatoes

- 4 cups vegetable broth

- 2 cans (14 oz each) black beans, drained and rinsed

- Salt and pepper to taste

- Chopped fresh cilantro for garnish

- Greek yogurt or sour cream for serving (optional)

Directions:

1. In a large saucepan, heat the olive oil over medium heat. Cook for approximately 5 minutes, or until the chopped onion has softened.

2. Add the minced garlic and simmer for another 1-2 minutes, or until fragrant.

3. Cook for 5 minutes, stirring in the chopped sweet potatoes, chili powder, ground cumin, smoked paprika, and cayenne pepper (if using).

4. Add the chopped tomatoes (with juices), vegetable broth, and black beans to the saucepan. Bring to a boil, then lower to a low heat and cook for 45 minutes to an hour, or until sweet potatoes are cooked.

5. Season with salt and pepper to taste.

6. Serve hot, topped with chopped fresh cilantro and a dollop of Greek yogurt or sour cream if preferred.

Nutrition Information (per serving):

- Calories: 250

- Total Fat: 3g

- Saturated Fat: 0.5g

- Cholesterol: 0mg

- Sodium: 800mg

- Total Carbohydrates: 45g

- Dietary Fiber: 12g

- Sugars: 10g

- Protein: 10g

Lemon Chicken Orzo Soup

Prep Time: 15 minutes
Cook Time: 30 minutes
Servings: 6

Ingredients:

- 1 tbsp. olive oil

- 1 onion, diced

- 2 carrots, diced

- 2 celery stalks, diced

- 2 cloves garlic, minced

- 1 lb boneless, skinless chicken breasts, cut into bite-sized pieces

- 6 cups chicken broth

- 1/2 cup uncooked orzo pasta

- 1 tsp. dried thyme

- Salt and pepper to taste

- Juice of 1 lemon

- Chopped fresh parsley for garnish

Directions:

1. In a large saucepan, heat the olive oil over medium heat. Cook for 5 minutes, stirring in the chopped onion, carrots, celery, and minced garlic.

2. Cook the bite-sized chicken pieces in the saucepan for 5 minutes, or until browned.

3. Stir in the chicken stock, uncooked orzo pasta, and dried thyme. Bring to a boil, then decrease heat to low and simmer for 15 minutes, or until the orzo is cooked through.

4. Season with salt and pepper to taste.

5. Add lemon juice immediately before serving.

6. Serve hot and garnish with chopped fresh parsley.

Nutrition Information (per serving):

- Calories: 250

- Total Fat: 5g

- Saturated Fat: 1g

- Cholesterol: 50mg

- Sodium: 800mg

- Total Carbohydrates: 30g

- Dietary Fiber: 3g

- Sugars: 5g

- Protein: 20g

Snacks

Avocado and Tomato Bruschetta

Prep Time: 10 minutes
Cook Time: 5 minutes
Servings: 4

Ingredients:

- 1 baguette, sliced
- 1 ripe avocado, mashed
- 1 cup cherry tomatoes, diced
- 2 tbsp. red onion, finely chopped
- 1 tbsp. fresh basil, chopped
- 1 tbsp. balsamic glaze
- Salt and pepper to taste

Directions:

1. Preheat the oven to 375° Fahrenheit (190° Celsius). Place the baguette pieces on a baking pan and bake for 5 minutes, until gently toasted.
2. In a bowl, combine mashed avocado, diced cherry tomatoes, red onion, and fresh basil.
3. Season with salt and pepper to taste.
4. Spoon the avocado mixture over toasted baguette pieces.
5. Drizzle with balsamic glaze before serving.

Nutrition Information (per serving):

- Calories: 150
- Total Fat: 6g
- Saturated Fat: 1g
- Cholesterol: 0mg
- Sodium: 200mg

- Total Carbohydrates: 20g

- Dietary Fiber: 3g

- Sugars: 2g

- Protein: 3g

Greek Yogurt with Honey and Almonds

Prep Time: 5 minutes
Servings: 1

Ingredients:

- 1/2 cup Greek yogurt

- 1 tbsp. honey

- 1 tbsp. almonds, chopped

Directions:

1. Spoon Greek yogurt into a serving dish.

2. Drizzle honey on the yogurt.

3. Sprinkle the chopped almonds over top.

4. Serve immediately.

Nutrition Information (per serving):

- Calories: 200

- Total Fat: 7g

- Saturated Fat: 1g

- Cholesterol: 10mg

- Sodium: 50mg

- Total Carbohydrates: 25g

- Dietary Fiber: 1g

- Sugars: 22g

- Protein: 12g

Baked Kale Chips

Prep Time: 10 minutes
Cook Time: 15 minutes
Servings: 4

Ingredients:

- 1 bunch kale, stems removed and leaves torn into bite-sized pieces
- 1 tbsp. olive oil
- Salt and pepper to taste

Directions:

1. Preheat the oven to 350° Fahrenheit (175° Celsius). Line a baking sheet with parchment paper.
2. In a large mixing bowl, combine the kale leaves, olive oil, salt, and pepper.
3. Spread the kale leaves in a single layer on the prepared baking sheet.
4. Bake in a preheated oven for 10-15 minutes, or until the kale is crisp but not browned.
5. Allow the kale chips to cool slightly before serving.

Nutrition Information (per serving):

- Calories: 50
- Total Fat: 3g
- Saturated Fat: 0g
- Cholesterol: 0mg
- Sodium: 100mg
- Total Carbohydrates: 5g
- Dietary Fiber: 1g
- Sugars: 0g
- Protein: 2g

Berry and Spinach Smoothie

Prep Time: 5 minutes
Servings: 1

Ingredients:

- 1 cup spinach leaves
- 1/2 cup mixed berries (such as strawberries, blueberries, raspberries)
- 1/2 banana
- 1/2 cup Greek yogurt
- 1/2 cup almond milk
- 1 tbsp. honey (optional)

Directions:

1. Combine spinach leaves, mixed berries, banana, Greek yogurt, almond milk, and honey (if using) in a blender.
2. Blend until smooth and creamy.
3. Pour into a glass and serve immediately.

Nutrition Information (per serving):

- Calories: 150
- Total Fat: 3g
- Saturated Fat: 0g
- Cholesterol: 5mg
- Sodium: 100mg
- Total Carbohydrates: 25g
- Dietary Fiber: 4g
- Sugars: 15g
- Protein: 8g

Quinoa and Black Bean Salad Cups

Prep Time: 15 minutes
Cook Time: 15 minutes
Servings: 4

Ingredients:

- 1 cup cooked quinoa
- 1 cup black beans, drained and rinsed
- 1 cup cherry tomatoes, halved
- 1/4 cup red onion, finely chopped
- 1/4 cup fresh cilantro, chopped
- Juice of 1 lime
- Salt and pepper to taste
- Lettuce leaves for serving

Directions:

1. In a large mixing bowl, add cooked quinoa, black beans, cherry tomatoes, red onion, and fresh cilantro.
2. Drizzle lime juice over the mixture and stir thoroughly.
3. Season with salt and pepper to taste.
4. Make cups out of lettuce leaves by spooning in quinoa and black bean salad.
5. Serve immediately.

Nutrition Information (per serving):

- Calories: 150
- Total Fat: 1g
- Saturated Fat: 0g
- Cholesterol: 0mg
- Sodium: 200mg
- Total Carbohydrates: 30g
- Dietary Fiber: 6g

- Sugars: 3g

- Protein: 7g

Apple Slices with Peanut Butter and Cinnamon

Prep Time: 5 minutes
Servings: 1

Ingredients:

- 1 apple, sliced

- 2 tbsp. peanut butter

- Pinch of ground cinnamon

Directions:

1. Arrange apple slices on a plate.

2. Spread peanut butter on each apple slice.

3. Sprinkle ground cinnamon over the peanut butter.

4. Serve immediately.

Nutrition Information (per serving):

- Calories: 250

- Total Fat: 16g

- Saturated Fat: 3g

- Cholesterol: 0mg

- Sodium: 120mg

- Total Carbohydrates: 25g

- Dietary Fiber: 6g

- Sugars: 16g

- Protein: 7g

Roasted Chickpeas with Garlic and Rosemary

Prep Time: 10 minutes
Cook Time: 40 minutes
Servings: 4

Ingredients:

- 2 cans (14 oz each) chickpeas (garbanzo beans), drained and rinsed
- 2 tbsp. olive oil
- 2 cloves garlic, minced
- 1 tbsp. fresh rosemary, chopped
- Salt and pepper to taste

Directions:

1. Preheat the oven to 400 °F (200 °C). Line a baking sheet with parchment paper.
2. Pat the chickpeas dry with a paper towel before spreading them out on the prepared baking sheet.
3. Drizzle olive oil over chickpeas and toss until evenly coated.
4. Sprinkle the chickpeas with minced garlic and chopped fresh rosemary, and season with salt and pepper to taste.
5. Roast the chickpeas in a preheated oven for 30-40 minutes, turning halfway through, until crispy and golden brown.
6. Allow the roasted chickpeas to cool slightly before serving.

Nutrition Information (per serving):

- Calories: 200
- Total Fat: 7g
- Saturated Fat: 1g
- Cholesterol: 0mg
- Sodium: 300mg
- Total Carbohydrates: 26g
- Dietary Fiber: 7g

- Sugars: 1g

- Protein: 8g

Whole Grain Crackers with Hummus and Cherry Tomatoes

Prep Time: 5 minutes
Servings: 1

Ingredients:

- Whole grain crackers

- Hummus

- Cherry tomatoes, halved

Directions:

1. Spread hummus onto whole grain crackers.

2. Top each cracker with a halved cherry tomato.

3. Serve immediately.

Nutrition Information (per serving):

- Calories: 150

- Total Fat: 5g

- Saturated Fat: 0.5g

- Cholesterol: 0mg

- Sodium: 200mg

- Total Carbohydrates: 20g

- Dietary Fiber: 4g

- Sugars: 2g

- Protein: 5g

Steamed Edamame with Sea Salt

Prep Time: 5 minutes
Cook Time: 5 minutes
Servings: 2

Ingredients:

- 2 cups frozen edamame in pods
- Sea salt for sprinkling

Directions:

1. Heat a kettle of water to a boil. Add the frozen edamame pods and simmer for 5 minutes.

2. Drain the edamame and transfer to a serving dish.

3. Sprinkle sea salt on the edamame pods.

4. Serve immediately.

Nutrition Information (per serving):

- Calories: 100
- Total Fat: 3g
- Saturated Fat: 0g
- Cholesterol: 0mg
- Sodium: 5mg
- Total Carbohydrates: 8g
- Dietary Fiber: 5g
- Sugars: 1g
- Protein: 9g

Cucumber and Feta Salad Skewers

Prep Time: 10 minutes
Servings: 4

Ingredients:

- 1 English cucumber

- 1/2 cup cherry tomatoes

- 1/2 cup feta cheese, cubed

- Fresh basil leaves

- Balsamic glaze for drizzling (optional)

- Toothpicks or skewers

Directions:

1. Cut cucumber into rounds approximately 1/2 inch thick.

2. Thread a cherry tomato, a cube of feta cheese, and a fresh basil leaf onto a toothpick or skewer.

3. Place the cucumber rounds on a serving dish and top with a skewer.

4. Drizzle with balsamic glaze if desired.

5. Serve immediately.

Nutrition Information (per serving):

- Calories: 50

- Total Fat: 3g

- Saturated Fat: 2g

- Cholesterol: 10mg

- Sodium: 100mg

- Total Carbohydrates: 3g

- Dietary Fiber: 1g

- Sugars: 2g

- Protein: 3g

Chia Seed Pudding with Mixed Berries

Prep Time: 5 minutes (plus chilling time)
Servings: 2

Ingredients:

- 1/4 cup chia seeds
- 1 cup almond milk (or any milk of your choice)
- 1 tbsp. honey (optional)
- 1/2 tsp. vanilla extract
- Mixed berries for topping

Directions:

1. In a dish, combine the chia seeds, almond milk, honey (if using), and vanilla essence.
2. Cover the bowl and refrigerate for at least 2 hours, or overnight, until the chia pudding is thick.
3. Stir the chia pudding before serving.
4. Spoon chia pudding into serving dishes and top with a variety of berries.
5. Serve cold.

Nutrition Information (per serving):

- Calories: 150
- Total Fat: 8g
- Saturated Fat: 1g
- Cholesterol: 0mg
- Sodium: 80mg
- Total Carbohydrates: 17g
- Dietary Fiber: 10g
- Sugars: 4g
- Protein: 4g

Roasted Red Pepper and White Bean Dip

Prep Time: 10 minutes
Cook Time: 25 minutes
Servings: 6

Ingredients:

- 1 can (15 oz) white beans (such as cannellini or Great Northern), drained and rinsed
- 1 jar (12 oz) roasted red peppers, drained
- 2 cloves garlic, minced
- 2 tbsp. olive oil
- Juice of 1 lemon
- 1/2 tsp. smoked paprika
- Salt and pepper to taste
- Fresh parsley for garnish

Directions:

1. Preheat the oven to 400 °F (200 °C).
2. In a food processor, mix the white beans, roasted red peppers, minced garlic, olive oil, lemon juice, smoked paprika, salt, and pepper.
3. Blend until smooth and creamy.
4. Transfer the dip to an oven-safe dish and bake for 20-25 minutes, or until hot and bubbling.
5. Garnish with fresh parsley before serving.
6. Serve with whole grain crackers, veggie sticks, or pita bread.

Nutrition Information (per serving):

- Calories: 150
- Total Fat: 6g
- Saturated Fat: 1g
- Cholesterol: 0mg
- Sodium: 300mg
- Total Carbohydrates: 19g
- Sugars: 1g
- Protein: 6g

Dessert

Berry Bliss Parfait

Prep Time: 10 minutes
Servings: 1

Ingredients:

- 1/2 cup Greek yogurt
- 1/4 cup mixed berries (such as strawberries, blueberries, raspberries)
- 2 tbsp. granola
- Drizzle of honey (optional)

Directions:

1. In a glass or dish, combine the Greek yogurt, mixed berries, and granola.
2. Repeat layering until all of the ingredients have been used up.
3. Drizzle honey over top if desired.
4. Serve immediately.

Nutrition Information (per serving):

- Calories: 200
- Total Fat: 5g
- Saturated Fat: 1g
- Cholesterol: 10mg
- Sodium: 50mg
- Total Carbohydrates: 30g
- Dietary Fiber: 3g
- Sugars: 15g
- Protein: 10g

Avocado Chocolate Mousse

Prep Time: 10 minutes
Servings: 2

Ingredients:

- 1 ripe avocado
- 2 tbsp. cocoa powder
- 2 tbsp. maple syrup or honey
- 1/2 tsp. vanilla extract
- Pinch of salt
- Optional toppings: berries, chopped nuts, shredded coconut

Directions:

1. Scoop the avocado flesh into a blender or food processor.
2. Combine cocoa powder, maple syrup or honey, vanilla essence, and salt.
3. Blend until smooth and creamy, scraping down the sides as necessary.
4. Divide the mousse into serving bowls.
5. Refrigerate for a minimum of 30 minutes before serving.
6. If preferred, add berries, chopped almonds, or shredded coconut.

Nutrition Information (per serving):

- Calories: 200
- Total Fat: 12g
- Saturated Fat: 2g
- Cholesterol: 0mg
- Sodium: 10mg
- Total Carbohydrates: 25g
- Dietary Fiber: 7g
- Sugars: 15g
- Protein: 3g

Lemon Chia Seed Pudding

Prep Time: 5 minutes (plus chilling time)
Servings: 2

Ingredients:

- 1/4 cup chia seeds
- 1 cup almond milk (or any milk of your choice)
- 2 tbsp. maple syrup or honey
- Zest of 1 lemon
- Juice of 1 lemon
- Optional toppings: lemon slices, berries, shredded coconut

Directions:

1. In a bowl, combine the chia seeds, almond milk, maple syrup or honey, lemon zest, and lemon juice.
2. Cover the bowl and refrigerate for at least 2 hours, or overnight, until the chia pudding is thick.
3. Stir the chia pudding before serving.
4. Divide the pudding into serving bowls.
5. Optional toppings include lemon slices, berries, or shredded coconut.

Nutrition Information (per serving):

- Calories: 150
- Total Fat: 7g
- Saturated Fat: 0.5g
- Cholesterol: 0mg
- Sodium: 80mg
- Total Carbohydrates: 20g
- Dietary Fiber: 7g
- Sugars: 10g
- Protein: 4g

Banana Oatmeal Cookies

Prep Time: 10 minutes
Cook Time: 15 minutes
Servings: 12

Ingredients:

- 2 ripe bananas, mashed

- 1 cup rolled oats

- 1/4 cup chopped nuts or seeds (such as walnuts, almonds, or sunflower seeds)

- 1/4 cup raisins or dried cranberries

- 1/2 tsp. cinnamon

- Pinch of salt

Directions:

1. Preheat the oven to 350° Fahrenheit (175° Celsius). Line a baking sheet with parchment paper.

2. In a mixing dish, add mashed bananas, rolled oats, chopped nuts or seeds, raisins or dried cranberries, cinnamon, and salt. Mix until well mixed.

3. Drop spoonfuls of the mixture onto the prepared baking sheet and shape them into cookies.

4. Bake the cookies in a preheated oven for 15 minutes, or until golden brown.

5. Allow cookies to cool for a few minutes on the baking sheet before moving them to a wire rack to finish cooling.

Nutrition Information (per serving, 1 cookie):

- Calories: 80

- Total Fat: 2g

- Saturated Fat: 0g

- Cholesterol: 0mg

- Sodium: 0mg

- Total Carbohydrates: 15g

- Dietary Fiber: 2g

- Sugars: 6g

- Protein: 2g

Dark Chocolate-Dipped Strawberries

Prep Time: 10 minutes
Cook Time: 5 minutes (for melting chocolate)
Servings: 12

Ingredients:

- 12 large strawberries, washed and dried

- 3 oz dark chocolate, chopped

- Optional toppings: shredded coconut, chopped nuts, sprinkles

Directions:

1. Line a baking sheet with parchment paper.

2. In a microwave-safe dish, melt the dark chocolate in 30-second increments, stirring in between, until smooth.

3. Dip each strawberry in the melted chocolate, allowing any excess to fall off.

4. Place the dipped strawberries on the prepared baking sheet.

5. Optional: Before the chocolate hardens, sprinkle the dipped strawberries with shredded coconut, chopped almonds, or sprinkles.

6. Refrigerate the strawberries for approximately 10 minutes, or until the chocolate hardens.

7. Serve cold.

Nutrition Information (per serving, 1 strawberry):

- Calories: 40

- Total Fat: 2g

- Saturated Fat: 1g

- Cholesterol: 0mg

- Sodium: 0mg

- Total Carbohydrates: 6g

- Dietary Fiber: 1g

- Sugars: 4g

- Protein: 0g

Greek Yogurt Fruit Salad

Prep Time: 10 minutes
Servings: 2

Ingredients:

- 1 cup Greek yogurt

- 1 cup mixed fruits (such as berries, diced apples, diced peaches)

- 2 tbsp. honey or maple syrup

- 1/4 tsp. vanilla extract

- Optional toppings: chopped nuts, shredded coconut

Directions:

1. In a bowl, blend Greek yogurt, mixed fruits, honey or maple syrup, and vanilla extract until thoroughly incorporated.

2. Divide the yogurt and berries into serving dishes.

3. If desired, add chopped nuts or shredded coconut on top.

4. Serve immediately.

Nutrition Information (per serving):

- Calories: 200

- Total Fat: 0g

- Saturated Fat: 0g

- Cholesterol: 5mg

- Sodium: 50mg

- Total Carbohydrates: 30g

- Dietary Fiber: 2g

- Sugars: 25g

- Protein: 17g

Almond Butter Energy Bites

Prep Time: 10 minutes
Chilling Time: 30 minutes
Servings: 12

Ingredients:

- 1 cup rolled oats

- 1/2 cup almond butter

- 1/4 cup honey or maple syrup

- 1/4 cup chopped almonds

- 1/4 cup shredded coconut

- 1/4 cup mini chocolate chips

- 1/2 tsp. vanilla extract

- Pinch of salt

Directions:

1. In a large mixing bowl, add rolled oats, almond butter, honey or maple syrup, chopped almonds, shredded coconut, micro chocolate chips, vanilla essence, and salt until thoroughly blended.

2. Roll the dough into tiny, 1 inch diameter balls and set them on a baking sheet lined with parchment paper.

3. Refrigerate the energy bites for a minimum of 30 minutes, or until firm.

4. Refrigerate in an airtight container for up to a week.

Nutrition Information (per serving, 1 energy bite):

- Calories: 150

- Total Fat: 8g

- Saturated Fat: 2g

- Cholesterol: 0mg

- Sodium: 20mg

- Total Carbohydrates: 16g

- Dietary Fiber: 2g

- Sugars: 9g

- Protein: 4g

Quinoa Berry Crumble

Prep Time: 10 minutes
Cook Time: 30 minutes
Servings: 6

Ingredients:

- 2 cups mixed berries (such as strawberries, blueberries, raspberries)

- 1 cup cooked quinoa

- 1/4 cup honey or maple syrup

- 1/4 cup almond flour

- 2 tbsp. coconut oil, melted

- 1 tsp. vanilla extract

- Pinch of salt

Directions:

1. Preheat the oven to 350° Fahrenheit (175° Celsius). Coat a baking dish with coconut oil or nonstick frying spray.

2. In a mixing bowl, add mixed berries, cooked quinoa, honey or maple syrup, almond flour, melted coconut oil, vanilla extract, and salt until thoroughly incorporated.

3. Transfer the berry mixture to the prepared baking dish.

4. Bake in a preheated oven for 25-30 minutes, or until golden brown and the berries bubble.

5. Let the crumble cool slightly before serving.

6. Serve warm with a dollop of Greek yogurt or a scoop of vanilla ice cream, if preferred.

Nutrition Information (per serving):

- Calories: 200

- Total Fat: 8g

- Saturated Fat: 4g

- Cholesterol: 0mg

- Sodium: 10mg

- Total Carbohydrates: 30g

- Dietary Fiber: 4g

- Sugars: 16g

- Protein: 3g

Coconut Mango Sorbet

Prep Time: 10 minutes
Freezing Time: 4 hours
Servings: 4

Ingredients:

- 2 ripe mangoes, peeled and diced

- 1/2 cup coconut milk

- 2 tbsp. honey or maple syrup

- Juice of 1 lime

- Pinch of salt

Directions:

1. Place the chopped mangoes in a blender or food processor.

2. Combine coconut milk, honey or maple syrup, lime juice, and salt.

3. Blend until smooth and creamy.

4. Transfer the mixture to a shallow dish or baking pan.

5. Freeze for one to two hours, or until the edges begin to freeze.

6. Remove from the freezer and use a fork to break up any remaining ice crystals.

7. Return to the freezer and continue every hour for 3-4 hours, or until the sorbet has set.

8. Serve sorbet in bowls or cones.

9. Enjoy right now.

Nutrition Information (per serving):

- Calories: 150

- Total Fat: 5g

- Saturated Fat: 4g

- Cholesterol: 0mg

- Sodium: 10mg

- Total Carbohydrates: 30g

- Dietary Fiber: 3g

- Sugars: 25g

- Protein: 1g

Baked Apples with Cinnamon

Prep Time: 10 minutes
Cook Time: 30 minutes
Servings: 4

Ingredients:

- 4 apples (such as Honeycrisp or Gala), cored

- 2 tbsp. honey or maple syrup

- 1 tsp. ground cinnamon

- Optional toppings: chopped nuts, raisins, Greek yogurt, granola

Directions:

1. Preheat the oven to 375° Fahrenheit (190° Celsius). Coat a baking dish with coconut oil or nonstick frying spray.

2. In a small dish, combine honey or maple syrup and ground cinnamon.

3. Place the cored apples in the prepared baking dish.

4. Drizzle the honey or maple syrup mixture over the apples, being careful to cover them evenly.

5. Bake in a preheated oven for 25-30 minutes, or until the apples are soft.

6. Remove from the oven and let to cool slightly before serving.

7. Optional toppings for baked apples include chopped nuts, raisins, Greek yogurt, or granola. Serve warm.

Nutrition Information (per serving):

- Calories: 150

- Total Fat: 1g

- Saturated Fat: 0g

- Cholesterol: 0mg

- Sodium: 0mg

- Total Carbohydrates: 40g

- Dietary Fiber: 6g

- Sugars: 30g

- Protein: 1g

Pistachio Cardamom Date Balls

Prep Time: 15 minutes
Servings: 12

Ingredients:

- 1 cup pitted dates

- 1/2 cup raw pistachios

- 1/2 tsp. ground cardamom

- Pinch of salt

- Optional coatings: shredded coconut, cocoa powder, crushed pistachios

Directions:

1. Place the pitted dates in a food processor and pulse until they create a sticky paste.

2. Put raw pistachios, ground cardamom, and a touch of salt in the food processor.

3. Pulse until the mixture is combined and the pistachios are finely chopped.

4. Scoop out tbsp.-sized amounts of the mixture and form into balls.

5. If preferred, roll each date ball with shredded coconut, cocoa powder, or crushed pistachios.

6. Refrigerate for a minimum of 30 minutes before serving.

7. Refrigerate in an airtight container for up to a week.

Nutrition Information (per serving, 1 date ball):

- Calories: 80

- Total Fat: 3g

- Saturated Fat: 0g

- Cholesterol: 0mg

- Sodium: 0mg

- Total Carbohydrates: 15g

- Dietary Fiber: 2g

- Sugars: 12g

- Protein: 1g

Blueberry Oat Bars

Prep Time: 10 minutes
Cook Time: 30 minutes
Servings: 12

Ingredients:

- 2 cups rolled oats

- 1 cup whole wheat flour

- 1/2 cup coconut oil, melted

- 1/2 cup maple syrup or honey

- 1 tsp. vanilla extract

- 1/2 tsp. cinnamon

- Pinch of salt

- 1 cup fresh or frozen blueberries

Directions:

1. Preheat the oven to 350° Fahrenheit (175° Celsius). Grease a 9-by-9-inch baking dish with coconut oil or nonstick cooking spray.

2. In a large bowl, combine the rolled oats, whole wheat flour, melted coconut oil, maple syrup or honey, vanilla essence, cinnamon, and salt.

3. Place half of the oat mixture in the bottom of the prepared baking dish.

4. Sprinkle the blueberries equally over the oat mixture in the baking dish.

5. Crumble the leftover oat mixture over the blueberries and press gently.

6. Bake for 25-30 minutes, until the top is golden brown and the blueberries are bubbling.

7. Allow the bars to cool fully in their baking dish before cutting into squares.

Nutrition Information (per serving, 1 bar):

- Calories: 200

- Total Fat: 8g

- Saturated Fat: 6g

- Cholesterol: 0mg

- Sodium: 10mg

- Total Carbohydrates: 30g

- Dietary Fiber: 3g

- Sugars: 12g

- Protein: 3g

Conclusion

The heart is a sign of love, yet the sad truth is that most people do not show their hearts the love they deserve. Consider the fact that heart disease is now the biggest cause of mortality. That is a frightening fact. However, by adopting preventative measures like eating a heart-healthy diet, you may increase your chances of overcoming the odds.

A healthy cardiac lifestyle may be enjoyable, tasty, and powerful, or it can seem burdensome and limiting. To succeed and have fun, evaluate the mentality you bring to this transformation. Then develop techniques to keep your motivation strong.

One method to help yourself is to practice mindfulness. Mindfulness is a means of paying attention to what you are feeling in the present moment. Beliefs like "I don't have time to care for myself with wholesome meals" or "I never make smart choices" may distract you from achieving your objectives; but, when you become aware of these very normal yet self-defeating thoughts, you have greater control over them. Self-compassion may help you break away from outdated patterns of thinking. Instead of instantly acting on those negative ideas, opt to veto them and choose a new path of action.

How does this work with eating? In this scenario, mindfulness allows you to acquire insight into how you speak to yourself and the impulses that drive your eating habits. This activity will help you break old habits and shift to meals that will keep you fuelled long-term. It will gradually become normal. Imagine how fantastic you'll feel after breaking old habits, achieving achievement, and improving your health! As time passes, your mindfulness practice will make you more conscious of how energetic and stable you feel when you nurture yourself in this manner. By taking the time to sit and enjoy your meal carefully, you may utilize mindful eating to check in with yourself whenever you eat. It becomes a more potent weapon as you practice it on a regular basis.

Thank you for reading this book. I wish you all the best!